Does Your Child Have Epilepsy?

James E. Jan, M.D., F.R.C.P. (C)
Clinical Professor, Division of Neurology, Department of Pediatrics
University of British Columbia
Seizure Clinic, Children's Hospital
Vancouver

Robert G. Ziegler, M.D.
Program Director, Family Service Team
Seizure Unit
Department of Psychiatry and Neurology
Children's Hospital Medical Center
Boston
and
Co-Director, Boundaries Therapy Center
Acton, Massachusetts

Giuseppe Erba, M.D.
Associate Professor in Neurology
Harvard Medical School
and
Associate in Neurology, Seizure Unit and
Division of Clinical Neurophysiology
Children's Hospital Medical Center
Boston

Does Your Child Have Epilepsy?

James E. Jan, M.D., F.R.C.P. (C)
Robert G. Ziegler, M.D.
and
Giuseppe Erba, M.D.

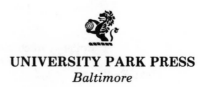

UNIVERSITY PARK PRESS
Baltimore

UNIVERSITY PARK PRESS
International Publishers in Science, Medicine, and Education
300 North Charles Street
Baltimore, Maryland 21201

Copyright © 1983 by University Park Press

Typeset by Oberlin Printing Company.
Manufactured in the United States of America
by The Maple Press Company.

This book was made possible through a grant
from Geigy Pharmaceuticals, U.S.A.

Library of Congress Cataloging in Publication Data

Jan, James E.
Does your child have epilepsy?

Includes index.
1. Epilepsy in children.   I. Ziegler, Robert G.
II. Erba, Giuseppe.   III. Title.
RJ496.E6J27   1982   618.92'853   82-15904
ISBN 0-8391-1758-2

Contents

Foreword by *E. R. Grass* ix
Preface xi
Acknowledgments xiii

Chapter **1** **What Does It Mean to Have a Child with Epilepsy?** 1
"He Is Our Child and We Love Him Dearly"
Epilepsy Is Common
Misconceptions
Must Epilepsy Be a Handicap?
Epilepsy Now And in the Past

Chapter **2** **What Is Epilepsy?** 11
The Brain Is a Marvelous Computer
What Is Epilepsy?
Common Terms
Why My Child?
Reaction to the First Seizure
What Brought the Seizure On?
Do Seizures Cause Brain Damage?
What Do I Tell My Young Child?
Starter Book

Chapter **3** **Tests Doctors Order** 31
Who Is the Best Physician to Treat a Child with Epilepsy?
History Taking
Examination
Brain Wave Test and the Preparation of the Child for It
The Interpretation of EEGs
X-rays and the CAT Scan
Blood Tests
Spinal Tap
Pneumoencephalogram and Angiogram
Hospitalization
References and Suggested Reading

Chapter **4** **Primary (Idiopathic) Generalized Epilepsy** 51
Absence Seizures (Petit Mal)
Convulsive Seizures (Grand Mal)
Light-Sensitive Seizures
Suggested Reading

Chapter **5 Partial and Secondary Generalized Epilepsy** 67
Partial (Focal) Epilepsy
Secondary Generalized Epilepsy
Differences and Similarities
Suggested Reading

Chapter **6 What is Not Epilepsy?** 89
Febrile Seizures
Hypnogogic Jerks, Twitches during Sleep,
   and Startling
Night Terrors
Migraine Headaches
Temper Tantrums
Daydreaming
Tics and Jerks
Fainting
Pallid Syncope
Breath-holding Spells
Psychogenic Epilepsy

Chapter **7 What Parents Should Know about Treatment** 103
How Drugs Work
How Medications Are Maintained
How Medications Are Started and Discontinued
Never Stop the Treatment on Your Own!
How Often Medications Need to Be Given
What If He Has Forgotten to Take His Pills?
Pills or Liquid?
Is My Child Going to Be An Addict?
Is an "Epileptic Always An Epileptic?"
What the Dentist Needs to Know
What Parents Need to Know about Pharmacies
Prescriptions
Why Parents Ask for A Second Medical Opinion
Both Parents Should Come for Appointments

Chapter **8 What Parents Should Know about Medications** 125
Selection of Medications
Side Effects
Measurements: Weight, Volume, and Length
Common Drugs and Their Side Effects
Where Should the Medication Be Kept?
When Medical Treatment Fails
Quack Advice
Protective Helmets
What to Do for Accidental Overdosage
How to Give Medications to an Uncooperative Child

Chapter **9 What to Do during a Convulsion** 145
How Parents Are Introduced to Epilepsy
Basic Rules
Important Observations during A Seizure
Should the Ambulance Be Called?
Should the Doctor Be Phoned?
How Can Long Seizures Be Stopped when Doctors and
   Hospitals Are Too Far Away?

Chapter **10**   **The Early Years** 155
Childhood Illnesses
Immunization
Babysitting
Identifying Chains and Bracelets
Sleeping Arrangements
Swimming and Bathing
Traveling
Entering School

Chapter **11**   **The Impact of Epilepsy:**
Common Feelings and Complications 163
The Child
Common Feelings
The Parents
The Siblings
The Family Network

Chapter **12**   **Adolescence and Young Adulthood** 175
Recreation, Sports, and Camping
Driving
Parties, Alcohol, Pot, and Smoking
Dating and Marriage
Pregnancy
Breastfeeding
Is Epilepsy Hereditary? Genetic Counseling
Insurance
Lay Epilepsy Organizations
The Rights of Children with Epilepsy in Education,
    Employment, and Health
Communication with Helpers
Suggested Reading

Chapter **13**   **The Multihandicapped** 187
The Burden of a Multihandicapped Child
Most Handicaps Are Not Readily Apparent at Birth
The Team Approach
Labels
Learning Difficulties
Hyperactivity
Mental Retardation
Cerebral Palsy
Visual and Hearing Impairment, Speech and Language Delay
Behavioral Problems
How to Use Limits to Help Children Grow and Learn
References

Chapter **14**   **Preparation for Work and Employment**
    —J. Lynne Mann, M.A., A.R.W. 203
Early Childhood
Elementary School Years
Transition to Secondary School
Secondary School Years
Preparation for the Job Hunt
Maintaining and Moving Up in Jobs
Summary of the Career Development Process

Where to Go for Help 219
Afterword 221
Index 223

Foreword

In 1908, Shelley wrote, in the *Dublin Review,*

"Know you what it is to be a child? It is to be something very different from the man of today. It is to have a spirit yet streaming from the waters of baptism; it is to believe in love, to believe in loveliness, to believe in belief; it is to be so little that the elves can reach to whisper in your ear; it is to turn pumpkins into coaches, and mice into horses, lowness into loftiness, and nothing into everything, for each child has its fairy godmother in its soul."

Such words exquisitely express universal hopes for the children in our care. How far removed from the grim realities that must be confronted by children with epilepsy and those who care for and about them. This book, *Does Your Child Have Epilepsy?,* gently bridges this significant gap with wisdom and loving kindness.

A foreword usually comments on relevance... therefore, the question: does epilepsy in children deserve a book of its own? Yes, enthusiastically, for both statistical and substantive reasons. About 30% of persons with seizures had the first one when they were less than 5 years old. Some 76% have had their first seizure experience by the age of 19. Epilepsy, therefore, is definitely a disorder of childhood.

Substantively, if we, with some difficulty, set aside the emotional impact of a child who has seizures, subtract our compassion, and try to examine childhood epilepsy strictly as a health problem, it makes sense pragmatically to treat seizures early in accordance with the axiom that early social and therapeutic intervention results in a more favorable outcome. We should not permit a child to acquire the seizure habit. This book provides material assistance.

Given that it is socially desirable and medically feasible to deal with seizures early, is the content of this book comprehensive? Does it deal with all of the important aspects of epilepsy? It is immediately obvious to the reader that the parents of children with epilepsy, and indeed the children themselves, have educated the authors in assembling the necessary and desirable subject matter. Because the authors have had fortunate access to numerically large and geographically diverse patient populations, the education has been extremely comprehensive and so is their presentation. The trio exemplifies Chaucer's philosophy, "For gladly would he teach, and gladly learn."

Writing a book of this sort presents certain tactical dilemmas. Parents are puzzled when the physician or social worker gives, an incomplete or indefinite answer to a direct question such as, "What caused my child's epilepsy?" Interpreting the state of the art in the field of epilepsy is far from simple. The authors are faced with how to give truthful, comprehensible answers; avoiding both oversimplification and overcomplication. For the most part, they have accomplished this goal honestly and well.

It is inevitable that there will be some who will disagree, for there is a plasticity at the fluid frontier of medical science and its companion technology that can be variably interpreted.

This is a very helpful, sensitively written book. Ten years ago the scene was vastly different. Ten years hence it will just as inevitably change, for "the human brain is the most complex structure in the known universe, so complex that it defies its own understanding."

The most important thing is that children continue *"to believe in loveliness,"* for as the book says, "They are our children and we love them dearly."

Ellen R. Grass, L.L.D.
Quincy, Massachusetts

Preface

When epilepsy is first diagnosed, the stunned parents often see it as a catastrophe striking the child and the whole family. They ask the same questions. Is she going to die? Is it due to a brain tumor? Will he be retarded? Is it our fault? Is epilepsy inherited?

At this stage, the physician cannot and should not attempt to explain all the pertinent facts on epilepsy and most parents are too upset to remember. But they soon recover and are starved for practical, comprehensive, and accurate information that has been written just for them. It is the role of health professionals to provide such material. This issue is so important that some epilepsy programs make parent education compulsory. This is not surprising, because the better parents and their children understand epilepsy, the more successful the treatment will be. Clearly, the management of a child with seizures is a shared responsibility between the parents and the health care providers.

Medications alone do not alleviate all the problems of children with epilepsy, a disorder which may affect so many aspects of their lives. Our book was written with these facts in mind but it does not replace the advice of physicians, nurses, social workers, psychologists, and others. On the contrary, we urge parents to ask more questions and expect answers.

We hope that the parents and the older child with epilepsy will benefit from reading this book. May we point out that throughout the text true case histories, with fictitious names, have been used.

In the management of children with epilepsy, parents must observe certain important principles. These basic rules, which are summarized below, will be mentioned frequently throughout the book.

**The Ten Basic Rules for Parents
Who Have Children with Epilepsy:**

1. *Collaboration*
   The responsibility of a child's treatment is shared between the parents and the physician.
2. *Trust*
   Parents and the older children need to develop a mutual trusting relationship with their doctor.
3. *Understanding*
   Family life is complex. Understanding means considering all the different factors and feelings which influence our choices.
4. *Knowledge*
   Understanding requires knowledge in order to be beneficial. Parents must learn about their child's epilepsy. This information and the physician's knowledge are both needed.
5. *Communication*
   It is often hard to explain problems, define solutions and communicate them. However, understanding and knowledge must be shared between doctor and family, parents and child.
6. *Medicine*
   Medications must be given regularly and should never be stopped abruptly without the physician's agreement.
7. *Rules*
   Rules and guidelines help a child mature and grow. They clarify complicated situations and make difficult problems easier to manage. They should be tailored to the needs of the child and the family. The parents should understand the doctor's rules and guidelines. Rules guard against overprotection.
8. *Love, Caring, and Cooperation*
   To cope with the child's epilepsy, the family together must nourish these feelings.
9. *Maintaining the Family Network*
   Other members of the family must not be neglected. Everyone has needs and a part to play. Parents should not isolate themselves and their child with epilepsy.
10. *Using Other Sources of Information*
    Families should use information and guidelines from different sources. These include social workers, nurses, educational specialists, EEG technicians, teachers, psychologists and psychiatrists, physical and occupational therapists, play therapists, and others.

James E. Jan
Robert G. Ziegler
Giuseppe Erba

Acknowledgments

Dr. Jan wishes to express his sincere gratitude, in alphabetical order, to the many individuals who offered their advice and so much of their time:

N. L. Auckland, M.D., Epileptologist; J. U. Crichton, M.D., Pediatric Neurologist; C. L. Dolman, M.D., Neuropathologist; H. G. Dunn, M.D., Pediatric Neurologist; K. Farrell, M.B., Epileptologist; J. Fletcher, R.N., Nurse Clinician; G. Gell, Photographer; Ellen R. Grass, L.L.D., Vice-Chairperson, Commission for the Control of Epilepsy and Its Consequences; F. Gray, Program Coordinator, Comprehensive Epilepsy Program, Minnesota; J. R. Hopkins, Executive Director, Vancouver Neurological Centre; Joan Johnson, Parent; J. Julian, R.N., Nurse Clinician; T. Martinez, R.N., Community Program Specialist, Comprehensive Epilepsy Program, Minnesota; L. Mitchell, Parent; R. Pearson, Parent; E. Powell, Parent; E. P. Scott, B.Ed., B.S.W., Social Worker; J. Srsen, Community Program Assistant, Comprehensive Epilepsy Program, Minnesota; J. A. Wada, M.D., Epileptologist.

This book would not have been written without the plight and inspiration of our little friends, Ryan, Linda, Seana, Jamie, Colin, and Jack, among others.

Dr. Ziegler's work at the Seizure Unit would not have been possible were it not for his introduction to epilepsy by Dr. Rysia Lombroso, as a result of her unflagging efforts for poor and handicapped children at Boston University's Division of Child Psychiatry. The second step was Dr. Cesare Lombroso's making a place for Dr. Ziegler on the staff of the Seizure Unit as part of his concern for the best treatment for children with seizures, including appropriate psychosocial diagnosis and care. Dr. Ziegler's colleagues on the Family Service Team, Cindy Ullman, Ellen Fishman, Betsy Broucek, and Lynn Holden have helped him survive the stresses of working with painful and difficult problems while enduring the adversities of a large medical/university complex. Dr. Giuseppe Erba and Dr. Valeria Cavazzuti extended his understanding of seizure disorders and neuropsychological functioning, rounded out by friendship and concern. Finally, his comprehension of the issues that most affect the lives of families, the men, women and children in them, was nurtured by the intimate tutelage of three: Patricia, Lisa, and Jeffrey. The other families who helped Dr. Ziegler learn most about the impact of seizures and brain dysfunction on individual and family functioning were the Spencers, Chris Accomando, Marty Fuller, George Janes, the Marcheses, and Karen Bourgeois.

Dr. Erba wishes to thank Charles F. Barlow, M.D., and Nancy Bassett for reviewing the manuscript.

The authors also wish to thank Ruby Richardson and Janet Hankin, Editors, and Debra Bass and Maureen McNeill, Production Editors of University Park Press, for their continuous advice and support.

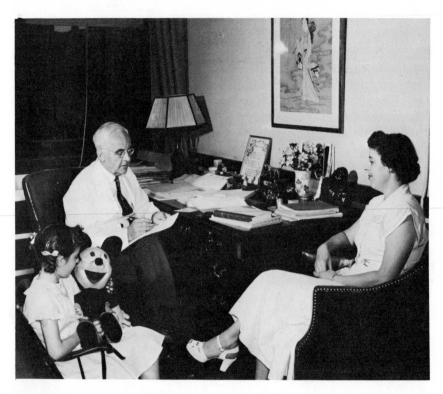

This book is a tribute to William G. Lennox, pioneer, scientist, innovator, and humanitarian who initiated the establishment of The Epilepsy Foundation of America and created the "model" for comprehensive care of children with epilepsy at the Boston Children's Hospital Medical Center. In the wake of Dr. Lennox's tradition, this book is dedicated to parents seeking knowledge and alliance to strengthen their fight against epilepsy.

Does Your Child Have Epilepsy?

chapter 1

What Does It Mean to Have a Child with Epilepsy?

"He Is Our Child and We Love Him Dearly"

Epilepsy Is Common

Misconceptions

Must Epilepsy Be a Handicap?

Epilepsy Now and in the Past

"He Is Our Child and We Love Him Dearly"

During the time this book was being written, the authors asked several parents for help. Their children had epilepsy, often with additional handicaps. In many cases, successful treatment was not readily obtainable.

The old saying that "the best teacher is your patient" is still true. Communication between children, their families, and physicians is beneficial to all concerned. Here are a few touching comments written by these parents on some aspects of epilepsy.

On the Diagnosis of Epilepsy

"It came as a hard blow because I had hoped it would not, could not be."

"That sort of thing happens to someone else."

"I thought it might be a symptom of a brain tumor. . . ."

"We have been so blessed by the prompt help we have received. Many people were not that lucky."

"We were shocked at the impotence of medical science. . . ."

On Attitudes Toward Epilepsy

"I told my parents, in-laws, and friends. They were stunned. One friend told me my son could never marry or have children. Later, I discovered that my husband's uncle had epilepsy; it had been a guarded secret."

"We had no problems with relatives or friends. They were so kind. . . ."

"His grandma expressed fears he was possessed. Others felt he should not marry. Others said he was faking it. Teachers thought he was lazy and inattentive."

"I think the thing that bothered me most was when people said, "Oh well, don't worry, he'll grow out of it."

"My family physician advised me not to tell my parents, relatives, friends, or school. The word epilepsy *was not to be used. These words*

reinforced my own fears, making me feel that epilepsy was a terrible thing, an unmentionable."

"We don't think that people are consciously prejudiced about children with seizures. They just watch and sometimes pass uneducated comments."

On Guilt Feelings

"I had taken some medication for a cold before I knew I was pregnant and worried about it for 9 months. Did this cause his epilepsy?"

"I was blaming myself for the problems he was having and wondered what I had done wrong during my pregnancy to cause them."

"We had no guilt feelings at all. The fact that our child's problem couldn't be traced to any genetic or prenatal cause made it easier."

On the Need for Appropriate Medical Information

"I couldn't find any information on epilepsy nor could I ask, since it was to be kept secret. All I had was the sketchy information in my home medical book. I did have a book printed in 1900, which stated epileptics were mentally ill and should be institutionalized when they became criminally violent."

"Phenobarb made him so lethargic that he sat in the gym and slept in class. I thought it was normal for anticonvulsants to do this—put him to sleep to stop seizures."

"The greatest fear of all was the damage the seizures would do to our child's body, perhaps even shortening his life span."

"Why isn't there more information for parents?"

On School

"The principal, after he found out the child had epilepsy, called me and asked me to take him home. I wouldn't; I told him he wasn't disturbing anyone."

"The teachers, not knowing he had epilepsy, would write that he was lazy and not trying."

"The teachers and everyone were most understanding. Everyone tried to help but they were too kind to her. This made her feel she was different."

On Their Children

"He gave his toys to his younger brother because he thought he was going to die. When he felt his attacks coming on he prayed: 'Please God don't let me have a seizure.' Sometimes the other children in the class also prayed."

"The other children in the family were very frightened and bewildered at what was happening to their little brother."

"It is hard to let a normal child "go" but even more difficult to do the same for an epileptic one."

On the Effect of Uncontrolled Seizures on Marriage and Social Life

"Fortunately, it has bound our marriage more firmly, as we don't blame each other regarding the problem. We understand each other's feelings and work together as a unit to help our son."

"Many families experience 'cabin fever.' Locked in, they are unable to get a break from constant stress of coping with a medical problem 24 hours a day. Marriages have broken up over it because home represents misery."

"Her health has had a profound effect on our social life, initially curtailing it completely. Our marriage at first suffered as a result of loss of expectations and freedom but later became stronger due to continued mutual efforts."

"Needless to say our social life suffered and still does. Very seldom do we get a chance to go out for an evening and when we do, we don't know what to do as we are so out of touch with the entertainment world."

"The seizures were controlled early and after a while we felt safe enough to leave her with a babysitter. Our social life was not affected."

On the Severely Multihandicapped Child

"Maybe it will come to institutionalization some day if we can't handle him but if and when it happens we can pat ourselves on the back for doing our best as parents instead of shrugging off the responsibility. He is our child and we love him dearly."

Advice to Other Parents

"Try not to be too frightened. Realize that you are not alone, it is not your fault and things will get better. Find out who the best specialist available is and see him quickly."

"Consider your child as a human being, that he or she belongs in society just as you do and fight for the child's rights."

Epilepsy Is Common

The incidence of epilepsy varies in different parts of the world. It occurs more frequently in developing countries because of malnutrition, infectious diseases, and inadequate medical care especially for pregnant women and babies. In the Western hemisphere approximately 1% of people have some type of epilepsy, and most of the time the first seizure occurs in childhood.

Epilepsy may seem to be rare until it affects a member of the family; then it is revealed that the boss in the office has a daughter with epilepsy, the neighbor down the road is taking anticonvulsant medications, a cousin had seizures as an infant, and someone's friend in school has staring spells. Epilepsy is common, and it affects anyone "with a brain" regardless of age, sex, or race.

Misconceptions

The problem is not just how little people know about epilepsy but that what they know is so often incorrect. Misbeliefs are common even among those with long-standing seizure disorders. Misconceptions determine how people with seizures react and cope with their condition; they can also increase the child's and family's burden of living with this disorder.

Here are some of the common incorrect answers to the question: What is epilepsy?

"An Epileptic Is Brain Damaged."

First of all, not all children with epilepsy have evidence of brain damage. Second, if the statement is true we must learn to interpret these two frightening words with caution and a realistic attitude. Brain damage is everything that has adversely affected the brain during development or later in life. At times it can be severe; other times it manifests itself as a subtle problem with coordination, speech, or learning. In Chapter 12, the difference between brain damage and brain dysfunction, or a delay in development, is discussed.

"Epileptics Are Retarded."

This is a very common misapprehension. Most individuals with epilepsy can be controlled on medications and become productive members in our society. Seizures are occasionally associated with brain damage; however, epilepsy by itself does not predispose individuals to mental retardation. In waiting rooms or in hospitals, the images of severely handicapped children with seizures may give the incorrect impression that epilepsy inevitably leads to brain damage. This association is a fact of life in some unfortunate cases, but it is certainly not the rule.

"Epileptics Are Mental."

Young friends, schoolmates, and even rather sophisticated adults think of this association when they witness the fearful expressions, loss of contact, automatic behavior, or aimless movements during the seizure of a child. Attention should be drawn to the fact that perceptual, mental, and motor functions return to normal upon termination of the attack. Of course, this does not mean that individuals with epilepsy cannot develop psychiatric illness like anyone else, or people with psychiatric disturbances cannot have seizures. The relationship between epilepsy and personality or mental disorders has been the object of dispute even among the medical profession. Some brain lesions that may cause seizures may also predispose persons to those disorders. This still largely unsettled issue is discussed in Chapter 2. One thing is certain: having seizures, no matter which type, is not synonymous with nor does it necessarily lead to mental illness.

"Most Criminals Are Epileptic."

Antisocial, sexual, and violent crimes in the past have been attributed to the epileptic personality without any scientific evidence to support this notion.

"Epileptics Should Never Get Married."

This is another incorrect belief. The issue of marriage is discussed in Chapter 12.

"An Epileptic Is a Person Who Swallows His Tongue during the Attack."

It is a common belief that an individual may swallow his or her tongue during an epileptic attack. This is physically impossible! When a child turns blue it is often because the muscles of respiration are affected by the seizure and the breathing may become shallow or can even stop for a short while. Accumulation of saliva or vomitus, however, may obstruct the respiration during a seizure. The gurgling or choking sound (often like someone with a snore) can be frightening and even dangerous. The proper handling of a child during an epileptic attack, described in Chapter 9, is easy to learn and easy to teach to others.

"The Saliva of an Epileptic Is Infectious and When It Is Smeared on a Baby, He May Get Epilepsy Later."

This idea originated from the Dark Ages in Europe and of course is totally false. A seizure is a complex symptom caused by a great variety of disturbances in the brain. It is not a disease. Occasionally an infectious illness such as meningitis or encephalitis may affect the brain, thus causing epilepsy. In no instances does the characteristic oversecretion of saliva occurring during epileptic attacks have a relationship to any infectious process.

"Epileptics Have Heart Attacks."

Occasionally heart attacks are confused with seizures, perhaps because during both afflictions a person may fall to the ground unconscious. Another common fear is that during a seizure the child's distress is so great that he or she may suffer a heart attack. This, however, is never the case.

"Epilepsy is the Work of the Devil."

This is a common belief in many Third World countries while the most common superstition in the West is that seizures mean such a person is crazy.

In television, radio, newspapers, schools, and in outpatient clinics, the public is being further educated about epilepsy. Today the misconceptions and prejudices are slowly diminishing. Education is one reason for this as well as the availability of more successful medical treatment.

Must Epilepsy Be a Handicap?

Disability is defined as a loss of an important function. Handicap refers to attitudes and feelings that turn disability into a problem of living. Individuals with uncontrolled seizures are disabled until they are successfully treated. When, however, they are restricted from certain activities and employment, cannot join athletic teams, are overprotected at home or in school, cannot drive cars, and so on, then they become handicapped. Because these disadvantages are often not readily apparent, epilepsy has justly been called an invisible handicap. Not only our society but also the parents, with their own attitudes and feelings, can handicap children with epilepsy even when their seizures are completely controlled. Many of these attitudes can be helped through appropriate education, and it is hoped that reading this book will show parents that the successful management of epilepsy is much more than just handing out medications.

Epilepsy Now and in the Past

Since ancient times, epilepsy has puzzled man. In one second the individual could be fine, and in the next he or she had fallen to the ground or was in a distant world. Most societies believed that gods or evil spirits "seized" the afflicted person; this explains the origin of the Greek word *epilepsy*. As long ago as 400 B.C., Hippocrates—the father of medicine—tried to dispel the common belief that epilepsy was a sacred disease. He argued that it was a disorder of the brain. The notion of epilepsy being a sacred disease continued, however, and became very popular in the Middle Ages. Cures were often attempted by religious means. Once the belief in spiritual possession was dispelled, other causes were imagined, and over the centuries bizarre diets, herbs, blood letting, induced sweating, and other useless forms of treatments were tried. There was no sure cure. For a long time epilepsy was believed to be infectious, spread mainly by saliva, and individuals with seizures were carefully avoided. One never ate from the dishes they used. Bizarre causes were considered. Moonlight was avoided because it could over heat or excessively cool the brain, thereby leading to epilepsy. Seizures were also believed to be caused by certain acts such as children under the age of 2 seeing their own image in the mirror or someone jumping over a lighted candle. Heredity was overemphasized. No wonder children with epilepsy and their families felt that this affliction had to be kept a secret.

The first therapeutic drug, bromide, was introduced in 1861 but it is no longer used because of the severe side effects. Then came phenobarbital in 1912, Dilantin in 1936, and a whole range of other medications. Electroencephalography as a clinical tool in the diagnosis of epilepsy was developed during the late thirties in Boston. Continuous advances are still being made. Thirty to forty years ago only a minority of people with epilepsy became seizure-free on treatment. Today, children with seizures have better diagnosis and care and a better chance of becoming productive members in our competitive society. The health profession is more interested in this disorder and research has markedly increased. Sophisticated epilepsy programs have emerged. Since the vast majority of seizures start in childhood, earlier diagnosis and intervention prevent a great many problems that might otherwise plague individuals in later life. Surgical techniques have been developed for the treatment of unremitting seizures. The attitudes of society toward epilepsy are more favorable. Laws have changed. Today, more emphasis is placed on what individuals with epilepsy can do than on what they can not do.

chapter 2

What Is Epilepsy?

The Brain Is a Marvelous Computer
What Is Epilepsy?
Common Terms
Why My Child?
Reaction to the First Seizure
What Brought the Seizure On?
Do Seizures Cause Brain Damage?
What Do I Tell My Young Child?
Starter Book

The Brain Is a Marvelous Computer

It may be useful to think of the brain as a complex computer that contains over 100 billion highly specialized cells (neurons) and intricate interconnecting pathways. Although the various parts of the brain carry out different functions, they work together in harmony like musicians in the finest orchestra. This awesome structure is still admired by scientists who study the innumerable aspects of its complexity and still do not understand it fully.

The formation of the central nervous system, (the brain and the spinal cord), begins within a few weeks after conception (Figure 1). This initial period is a sensitive stage for the rapidly developing embryo, because even mildly noxious substances may hurt it. Excessive alcohol, heavy smoking, drugs, virus infections, and other maternal illnesses may affect this delicately budding structure. The fetus becomes more resistant to insults of that sort after 3 to 4 months. At birth when the umbilical cord is cut, the newborn passes once more through critical changes from being totally dependent on the mother's body to a more autonomous existence. The infant now requires parental care. Most neurons are formed by this time but they continue to grow in size and specialize throughout the first 10 years of life. Likewise, the various interconnecting pathways do not fully mature until the end of the first 2 decades.

The maturation of this marvelous computer allows the child to learn and master various actions and ideas at different times. The 6-month-old is busy acquiring the balance, strength, and coordination needed to sit, while the 6-year-old uses them for riding a bicycle. The brain is a functional unit with varying balances of strengths and weaknesses. For example, excellent artists or scientists can be poor readers. In other words, whereas the so-called normal individual is expected to perform evenly in all areas, superior abilities in certain functions may be associated with other inferior ones.

The way the brain works is extremely complex and the manifestations of epilepsy are tied up with this complexity. Therefore, par-

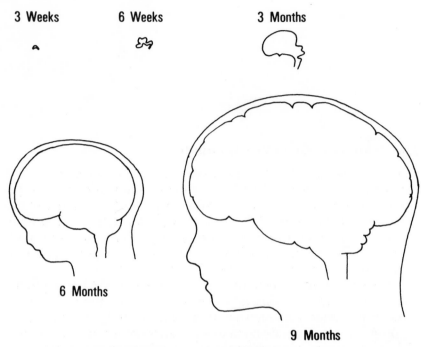

3 Weeks   **6 Weeks**   **3 Months**

6 Months

9 Months

Figure 1.   The development of the human brain from conception to birth.

ents need to learn where fundamental functions are performed, in order to understand where seizures are thought to originate and why they present certain symptoms (characteristics). The upper part of the brain (the cerebrum) is divided into two halves (the hemispheres) (Figure 2, Figure 3, Figure 4). They contain grey and white matter. The grey matter consists of millions of neurons disposed in layers and orderly columns. The brain is covered with a superficial ribbon of grey matter (the cortex) and several islands lie deep underneath. The rest of the hemispheres is white matter, which represents the massive hardware wiring to innumerable connective pathways between individual and groups of cells. The brain as seen from the surface, contains distinct regions: the frontal, parietal, temporal, and occipital lobes. All have recognized functions. For example, the cortex of the occipital lobe receives visual information, whereas sound and speech are recorded in the temporal lobes. The frontal lobes are responsible for initiation of voluntary movements, they integrate complex motor activity, and they control several important aspects of behavior. The parietal lobes are involved in decoding sensations coming in from all parts of the body (inputs). They also function as a

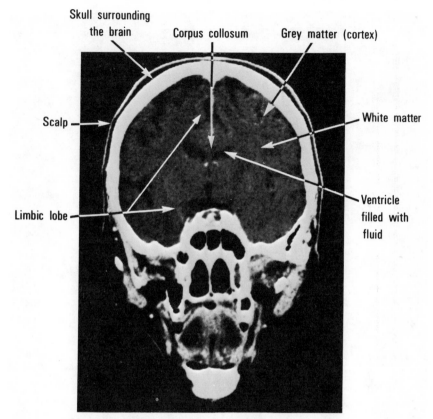

Figure 2.   A cross-section of the brain as seen in a CAT scan.

highly sophisticated feedback system to increase the efficiency of
the motor responses (outputs). Because of their central location, the
parietal lobes integrate body sensations with visual and auditory
input received in the occipital and temporal lobes. Such combined
information is then relayed to the frontal lobes. Each hemisphere as
a whole and each lobe individually is communicating with the other
on the opposite side through a large, thick bundle of white matter
(corpus callosum). The portion of cortex that lies all around this major interconnecting pathway, the limbic lobe (Figure 2), represents
the most primitive but a very important part of the brain. It is involved in the coordination of lower level functions, such as consolidation of memory, visceral (deep) sensations and motility, automatic regulation of blood pressure, heart rate, gland secretion,
emotions that do not require conscious and voluntary intervention.

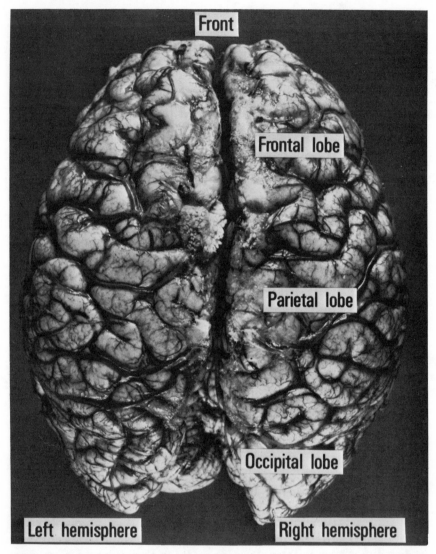

Figure 3.   The brain viewed from above. Each part of this "computer" serves a different function.

Physicians frequently point out in simple terms that the right side of the brain controls the left side of the body. (This is not true for the limbic cortex where specialization and lateralization are not as developed as in other lobes.) Although they look alike, functionally the two hemispheres are not identical. Gradually, in the first few

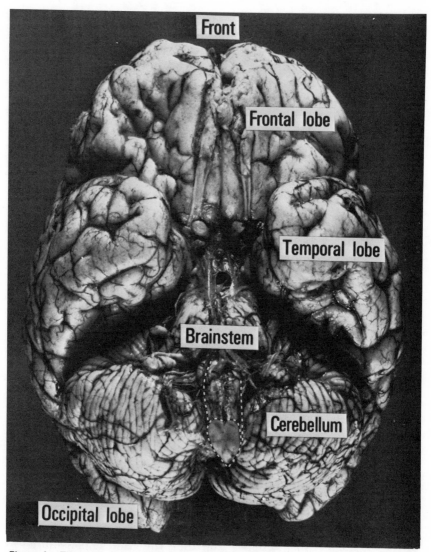

Figure 4. The brain viewed from below. The lowest part of the brainstem, the medulla is outlined by a dotted line. It was severed from the spinal cord.

years of life, one becomes dominant over the other. This process is closely connected with the development of handedness. When a child is right-handed, the left hemisphere is defined as dominant because it is in this half of the brain where important forms of communication such as language skills are located. In a left-handed child the opposite may be true. The nondominant hemisphere specializes in equally important skills such as perception of space and orientation. The white matter pathways connecting the hemispheres with the spinal cord join in the brain stem (Figure 4). Here is a central core of grey matter that regulates sleep, waking, and the state of alertness (or readiness to perform) of the individual. When seizure discharges involve this region, a loss of consciousness is expected. Because each area of the brain has distinct functions and the interconnecting pathways are known, the neurologist can often predict and identify the site of the disturbance by relating the pattern of the seizures to these anatomical structures. This will then determine which diagnostic tests are required.

What Is Epilepsy?

A seizure can occur at any age. It is usually a brief, sudden malfunction of the brain that is attributable to a massive abnormal electrical discharge. During these episodes the electroencephalogram (EEG) can record abnormal electrical activity (Chapter 3). What the child does during the seizure depends a great deal on where in the brain this disturbance is. For example, when the occipital lobe is involved, the child may "see" brightly colored spots before his or her eyes, or when twitching of one arm occurs, the corresponding motor area on the opposite side of the brain is affected. Although the appearance of the discharge in the EEG can greatly vary, a seizure is but a symptom of this electrical trouble in that particular region of the brain.

Although the words *seizure* and *epilepsy* are often used interchangeably, not all seizures are epileptic in nature. A seizure is not "epilepsy" when it is the result of another physical problem. For example, low blood sugar or a severe infection can cause an electrical disturbance in the brain, thereby a seizure; still, the child does not have epilepsy. On the other hand, when the seizures recur, unpredictably and without another medical reason, this constitutes a medical entity in itself called epilepsy and then the child is considered to have an epileptic seizure disorder.

Common Terms

Eileen Fast had received anticonvulsant treatment for her seizures for years, but her family physician had never mentioned epilepsy. When she was referred to the clinic the parents were quite upset following the remark that their daughter had epilepsy. "We did not know she was an epileptic. How could Dr. Williams miss the diagnosis? If he knew, why didn't he tell us? We are shocked!" Eileen's doctor knew she had epilepsy but he had simply used another term, *seizure disorder* without specifying the nature.

The epileptic attack is often described by many different words, such as seizure, fit, convulsion, blackout, spell, episode, shakes, and nervousness. Children may create their own descriptive terms like "dizzies," "shakies," and "falls." The difference between epilepsy and seizures has already been pointed out. A convulsion is a type of seizure during which the person's whole body shakes in contrast to a staring spell when the individual simply becomes momentarily unaware but does not fall. A blackout is more like fainting than a seizure. Most of us know enough French to realize that *grand* means big and *petit* means small. *Grand mal*, however, does not describe a big (severe) seizure, nor does *petit mal* describe a small (slight) one. In medical terms *grand mal* indicates a generalized convulsion starting with stiffening of the body (tonic phase) followed by rhythmic contractions (clonic phase) associated with a transient period of unconsciousness. In *petit mal* only a brief period of unresponsiveness occurs. In *focal* (partial) seizures the electrical disturbance is limited to one area, whereas in *generalized* seizures the whole brain is involved. A seizure may start focally (in one small area) in the cortex of one hemisphere, then spread and become secondarily generalized. Because epilepsy can take on so many forms, and the underlying process is still poorly understood, the classification of seizure disorders is difficult. Some types of focal epilepsy are named after the region they most commonly originated from, as for example, frontal, parietal, temporal, and occipital lobe seizures. Because there is a great deal of overlap in the site of origin these terms should be replaced with ones that describe the symptoms more strictly. To achieve more uniformity in describing the different seizure patterns, an international classification system recently was developed. Its detailed description is beyond the scope of this book, but whenever possible the new international terminology is used. During a child's treatment, many medical words are mentioned that may sound unfamiliar to parents. Parents must ask their physicians to explain the medical terminology. They should also remember that the first five rules for epilepsy are collaboration, trust, understanding, knowledge, and communication.

On the other hand some of the above terms originated in times when epilepsy was considered to be an incurable and disastrous affliction. It is not surprising, therefore, that they have developed negative connotations. Nevertheless, the condition should be called what it is. When parents feel uneasy with the word *epilepsy*, it is a clue that they are facing the medical problem with less than a realistic attitude. Discussing these feelings with the doctor, or another helper, may be very beneficial. When we understand our anxieties it is easier to obtain new information about our problems or solve them.

Why My Child?

When epilepsy occurs in a family, parents feel bewildered and wonder why it has happened to their child. The answer may or may not be obvious. Whatever the reason, sadness or even anger are common feelings.

> Julie was a second child. Her mother had had frequent small vaginal bleeds, stomach cramps, and poor health during the first few months of pregnancy. In the middle trimester, she developed repeated kidney infections, was hospitalized and treated with antibiotics. At the end of her pregnancy her blood pressure was high and she began accumulating excess fluid in her body. Julie was then born 6 weeks early. She weighed less than 3 lbs.; by calculation, she should have been 5 lbs. Julie's first seizure occurred at just 12 hours of age, and she had more seizures later in spite of adequate anticonvulsant therapy. Her physician diagnosed epilepsy as a result of brain damage occurring during the abnormal pregnancy. The baby's tests showed a severely damaged small brain."

Health problems during pregnancy, especially in the early months when the embryo is rapidly growing, can be very damaging to the developing brain. This is why proper maternal health care is so important.

> Mrs. Norden's pregnancy was seemingly normal but her little boy was born with multiple deformities. The infant had frequent seizures and died at 2 days of age. Tests revealed that his maldevelopment was due to a chromosomal abnormality.

Chromosomal abnormalities are a rare cause of seizures and they are suspected when an infant is born with multiple defects. The progress in medical sciences has not eliminated these disasters that cause unusual and heart rending experiences. These are times when parents need each other, their family network, and often, someone outside the family to whom they can talk. Talking cannot alter the facts but it can help us understand our feelings better and permit us to manage as best as possible.

Frequently there is no obvious explanation why a child has epilepsy. The pregnancy, birth, and subsequent development were normal and no one in the family ever had seizures. Investigations in such children may turn out to be entirely negative (normal). This is true in over half the cases. The doctor will call this an idiopathic case, meaning that the underlying cause is, for the time being, not known. Parents often find this difficult to accept because "there just has to be a reason and when it is known the remedy can be found." Even when the cause is known there are diseases such as the common cold, which is due to viruses, where we still have to suffer through our aches, pains, and sniffles. As another example, although the cause of diabetes is understood, still regular medications and continuing collaboration between physician and family are required.

As discussed above, the brain contains over 100 billion neurons, and when only a small area is disturbed, all the tests may still be "normal." In fact, when the investigations are negative, the prognosis is generally better for complete seizure control and treatment is usually easier. However, it is understandable that parents feel frustrated by the lack of an explanation and are made more apprehensive by this uncertainty. The doctor will continue to "look" for a cause.

In a very small number of children, a brain tumor is responsible for the seizures. Fortunately, this happens rarely but parents often fear this possibility. In the majority of cases these brain tumors are benign and are treatable by surgery and/or radiation. They need to be removed because, although slow-growing, they cause compression of the brain and eventually cause worsening of the seizures and neurological deficits. These tumors may be present from birth and may not be detectable at the onset of the seizure disorder. This is an example where the "cause" of epilepsy is initially not detected (cryptogenic). (*Idiopathic* is another term for unknown.) If a cause eventually is found it may be removed. This means that every cryptogenic case must be routinely re-examined.

There are also epileptic children with a strong family history of seizures. The genetic factors responsible have been extensively studied but are still poorly understood. This topic is discussed in Chapter 12.

Head injury is another possible cause of epilepsy. Usually, traumas need to be quite severe before they can produce damage leading to epilepsy. There are two types of head trauma: open and closed. An open head injury with depressed and fragmented fractures of the skull, laceration of the membrane surrounding the brain (the dura) and loss of the underlying brain substance, carries the greatest risk for developing a seizure disorder. In a closed head trauma the brain may be bruised by the violent impact against the bone ridges inside the skull. These bruises could lead to scar tissue which may eventually be the cause of an epileptic disorder. A *concussion* implies loss or alteration of consciousness after the trauma with loss of memory of the event. A simple concussion does not carry a great risk of epilepsy. The doctor will inquire, however, about the severity of these symptoms. The more violent the impact on the head, the greater is the concussion and the possibility of also having bruises on the brain, which may lead to seizures.

In *"post-traumatic"* epilepsy there is usually a gap of 6–24 months between the head trauma and the onset of seizures. That is why preventive treatment with anticonvulsants during this period is often advised even if no seizures have occurred. A simple linear skull fracture (a hairline crack in the skull) usually does not carry risk of epilepsy unless there is evidence of concussion and the possibility of having bruised the brain.

Other causes of epilepsy include lack of oxygen at birth; infectious diseases, such as meningitis, encephalitis or brain abscess; intoxications (such as lead or mercury poisoning); inherited or degenerative central nervous system disorders or strokes. These can all lead to seizures.

Parents should not be afraid to discuss their doubts and fears about possible causes of the seizures affecting their child. They often have hidden guilt feelings due to real or imaginary causes even if the doctor may not have all the definite answers. Such feelings must come out because conflicts must be resolved; otherwise they may interefere with the family life and the child's care.

Reaction to the First Seizure

Epilepsy can affect anyone, at any age, but most commonly it appears in childhood (Figure 5). Parents are often puzzled by why epilepsy surfaces months, or even years after a difficult birth, an accident, an episode of meningitis, or even without an apparent cause. Sometimes an explanation can be found, at other times it is not clear. In general, it is not the loss of neurons at the time of brain injury that causes the seizures but rather the development of scar tissue at the site of the injury. This takes time to be formed.

When parents learn that their child has epilepsy, they first must respond to the reality of the situation. This means obtaining proper and necessary medical attention. It may also mean looking for an

AGES WHEN EPILEPTIC SEIZURES FIRST OCCUR

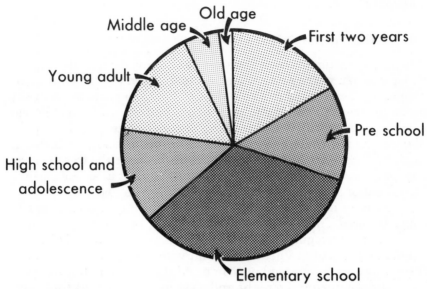

Figure 5. Most commonly the first epileptic seizure occurs in childhood.

opportunity to discuss things with a counselor who can be the family physician, a neurologist, a nurse, a social worker, or someone else. A frantic search from doctor to doctor, clinic to clinic, for a "cure" should be avoided. Thinking and talking things through can help in facing the situation. Parents should never search for a miracle but for the best and most sensible care.

Few parents are prepared to deal emotionally or intellectually with the news that their child has epilepsy. Even those who have a professional background (which may even include familiarity with seizure disorders) experience the natural sense of shock and dismay. Feelings can become troublesome when they get in the way of appropriate action in the child's behalf. If the only outcome of shock is doubt, inability to cope, a sense of defeat or resentment, our emotions are no longer at work for us. Once we can clearly acknowledge and deal with a sense of hurt, grief or dismay, the better we will be able to manage our predicament. Parents, therefore, will require much support. They need not be afraid to ask for support and to search for information. The less informed they are, the more likely they are to become the victims of emotional and irrational reactions to the diagnosis of epilepsy. The basic rule of knowledge (learning about epilepsy) also means learning to deal with epilepsy. This is as important for a parent as it will be later in life for the child who experiences a seizure disorder.

What Brought the Seizure On?

When a youngster has been diagnosed as having a particular form of epilepsy, seizures may return unexpectedly, even when the medicine seems to provide good control. Most of the time parents naturally probe for reasons and try to establish a pattern. Did the child eat something harmful? Was it teething or constipation? Did he or she play too hard? Too much sunshine? Perhaps a cold, tiredness, or anxiety? These are all sensible questions because the treatment of epilepsy does not only consist of medications but also includes the identification and prevention of precipitating factors.

Certainly inadequate treatment and missing medications can cause seizures. This is discussed in Chapter 7. In general, variations in the diet, or irregular meals do not bring on epilepsy. Too much sunshine, exposure to heat, cold, and wind are rarely significant. Sleep, however, seems to play an important role. Some children have their attacks during the night and daytime naps. Night time (nocturnal) seizures tend to occur either shortly after falling asleep (deep sleep) or early in the morning before waking (light sleep). Excessive drowsiness may also precipitate epileptic attacks. When children with epilepsy go to bed later than usual and the next day are very tired they could have a seizure. It must be stressed, however, that they need adequate, not extra sleep.

Teething and constipation in infants are often blamed for triggering seizures; there is little scientific proof of this, although stress, which accompanies such situations, may be an influencing factor. Some children may have flurries of seizures during a febrile illness. Seizures can be precipitated by flickering light, as for example, when a car or a train passes through trees. A flickering TV (changing channels or adjusting the image) may cause a convulsion if the child is photosensitive. Emotional pressure, fatigue, feeling of inadequacy, and excessive anxiety may trigger epileptic attacks. In most instances there is no obvious precipitating cause. Parents should bring up the issue of possible triggering factors with their doctor.

Do Seizures Cause Brain Damage?

Caroline had absence seizures (petit mal) and was 6 years old when she was first seen at the seizure clinic. Her mother tearfully confessed that she had lost all hope for her child's recovery. Almost a year before, when the diagnosis was made, she asked her physician if treatment was necessary. He answered that it was important because seizures can cause brain damage. The doctor probably meant big seizures with impairment of breathing but this was not made clear to the parents. This dreadful "fact" was made worse by a close family friend stating that every time someone had a seizure, many brain cells were destroyed. Although the medications, with periodic adjustments, had greatly helped Caroline's seizures, she still had the occasional staring spell. Her terrified parents helplessly watched their daughter becoming "brain damaged." They felt such constant fear that the last 12 months were almost unbearable. While the medications needed only minor adjustments, what the parents really needed was time to talk comfortably with someone who would listen and then provide some accurate information. The parents were assured that generally, only prolonged and difficult seizures might cause brain damage. Nine years later Caroline was a top student in her freshman class in high school. Because she had been seizure free for 5 years, the medications were discontinued without any problems.

Unfortunately, it is a common belief among the public, and even among health professionals that seizures inevitably lead to brain damage. Perhaps the cause of this misconception is manifold. First of all there are children with rare untreatable, progressive neurological diseases who also have seizures and gradually deteriorate physically and mentally, and finally die. It is not their epilepsy that leads to deterioration and death but the underlying uncontrollable illness. Seizures are symptoms of their brain disorder, and it is the underlying process that may or may not produce damage. Relatives and friends often do not realize this. Second, during certain prolonged convulsions, the metabolic demands of the neurons involved in the electrical discharge may be so high that these cells become vulnerable. It is accepted by most neurologists that only long uncontrolled seizures, lasting not for minutes but for hours (status epilepticus) may cause damage to the neurons. The immature brain of newborns seems to be more vulnerable to the insult of prolonged seizures than it is later in life. Since the brain has billions of cells, how many lost neurons will result in significant "brain damage?" Although this is still a controversial issue, it can be stated with confidence that in the great majority of recurrent seizures, even major tonic-clonic convulsions, are followed by complete clinical recovery.

What Do I Tell My Young Child?

First, what should a toddler or a preschool child be told? This exercise is important because it is the first step in building their participation in self-care and future responsibilities. Helping children to grow is built on trust and on our understanding of them. Parents should, therefore, communicate their knowledge. It is important to remember that young children have different concerns than those that worry adults. Children should be comfortable with the present situation, need to be prepared for different experiences, and above all, must feel safe. At this stage they accept the spells as part of their "normal" existence as they cannot comprehend the complex consequences of a seizure disorder.

Parents must spend adequate time preparing their children for the experiences resulting from meeting doctors and other health professionals. Together they can write a book about the different aspects of the medical examination. As they grow older, more and more information can be included. It can be read for a bedtime story (a week's repetition is a good start to ensure familiarity with each idea). It may also be an aid for "doctor play" during the day. Pages can be added in a scrap book like fashion for special medical events and for when they begin to describe their own observations regarding their seizures and treatment.

Starter Book

Page 1   The first project is the title and the decoration of the front page.

Page 2   THE DOCTOR USES

EYES

EARS

AND HANDS

TO LEARN ABOUT THE BODY

(Pictures of eyes, ears and hands are cut and pasted here. These can also be drawn simply by the parents or children.)

Page 3   EYES TO LOOK AT FINGERS AND TOES

EYES TO LOOK IN MOUTHS

EYES TO LOOK AT EYES

EYES TO WATCH US SIT, WALK, AND SKIP

Page 4   EARS TO HEAR US BREATHE

EARS TO HEAR OUR HEART

EARS TO HEAR US COUGH

Page 5   HANDS TO FEEL

LET'S FEEL OUR HEADS

LET'S FEEL OUR CHESTS AND OUR TUMMIES

LET'S FEEL HOW STRONG OUR MUSCLES ARE

LET'S FEEL SOMETHING SHARP

(Practice with a toothpick)

SOMETHING SOFT AND FUZZY

(Use a cotton ball)

COLD AND HARD

(Use a spoon)

(Sometimes children will be more interested in these activities than others and they should be allowed to go at their own pace.)

Page 6 ## THE DOCTOR HAS HELPERS JUST THE WAY MOM AND DAD HELP YOU

THE DOCTOR USES A LIGHT

(Practice shining a light in eyes, ears, mouth, and at toes and tummy.)

THE STETHOSCOPE IS ALSO A DOCTOR'S HELPER, SO IS A RUBBER HAMMER.

(A doctor's toy kit could be used. The child can play with it when the book is read and when alone.)

Page 7 ## THE DOCTORS HAVE HELPERS THAT ARE MACHINES

MACHINES CAN TAKE PICTURES

(Cut and paste a camera)

MACHINES LIKE THE EEG MACHINE CAN TELL ABOUT OUR HEAD

(See the section on the brain wave test in Chapter 3)

Page 8 ## THE EEG MACHINE WORKS LIKE THIS

(The child holds three different colored crayons together to draw squiggly lines. At the EEG test, a sample of the record can be obtained.)

THE DOCTOR'S HELPER MAKES MARKS ON YOU

(A washable magic marker can be used to draw little "x's" on the body, on the cheeks, and forehead of the child. The technicians will make marks only on the head for accurate placement of the electrodes.)

THEN THE DOCTOR'S HELPER PUTS ON SPOTS

(Spot stickers from the store can be used by the children to stick on their bodies when they have made a mark.
The EEG technicians put tiny electrodes over the marks.)

Page 9 DOCTORS SOMETIMES USE NEEDLES.

NEEDLES ARE SHARP. THEY CAN MAKE US SAY OUCH, AND CRY.

HOLDING STILL FOR THE NEEDLES IS A BIG JOB. IT IS HARD TO DO. MOM OR DAD CAN HELP.

NEEDLES CAN MAKE US MAD.

Page 10 JUST LIKE YOU AND ME, THE DOCTOR USES EYES, EARS AND HANDS TO FIND OUT ABOUT THINGS.

THE DOCTOR WILL TELL WHAT HE LEARNED ABOUT US.

HE WILL HELP US KEEP WELL.

(A picture of a doctor can be pasted or drawn.)

If the child is between the ages of five and ten years, the same book can be written at the appropriate level. Trips to the library are a good way to find out about physicians and hospitals. More information about each test, the epileptic attacks and the way the brain and body work may be included. The subject of discussing seizures with the school age child and the adolescent will follow the descriptions of different seizure disorders in Chapters 4 and 5.

chapter 3

Tests Doctors Order

Who Is the Best Physician to Treat
  a Child with Epilepsy?

History Taking

Examination

Brain Wave Test and the Preparation of
  the Child for It

The Interpretation of EEGs

X-rays and the CAT Scan

Blood Tests

Spinal Tap

Pneumoencephalogram and Angiogram

Hospitalization

References and Suggested Reading

Who Is the Best Physician to Treat a Child with Epilepsy?

Although most doctors are familiar with epilepsy some specialize in this field. A family physician treats many different types of illnesses, which requires wide-spread knowledge. A pediatrician has more training in seizure disorders, but not as much as a neurologist, (who treats disorders of the nervous system), particularly a pediatric neurologist. A few doctors, epileptologists, restrict their practice to epilepsy and work in seizure clinics, mostly those attached to large medical centers.

When the seizures are easily controlled, parents may stay under the care of their family physician or pediatrician. It is still advisable, however, to obtain at least one consultation from a trained specialist. For the treatment of a child with a difficult form of epilepsy, pediatric neurologists, epileptologists, or seizure clinics in a pediatric hospital are the best choices. Unfortunately for many families, the major medical centers, where highly trained specialists usually practice, are often far away. A single consultation, however, might be worth the effort, particularly in complicated cases.

Parents need to feel comfortable with their doctor and develop a mutual trust, without which treatment is often less successful. When they choose their physician, they should remember that a very busy practice does not always offer the best care. The treatment of seizure disorders requires time for discussion and a working partnership between the doctor and the parents.

History Taking

When a child with a seizure disorder is referred to a specialist, a careful history is obtained. Seemingly endless questions are asked regarding the pattern of seizures, pregnancy, birth, early development, education, academic achievement, behavior, health, injuries, and even about the other members of the family. The physician begins to formulate answers to important questions: Was that episode

really epilepsy? What part of the brain was affected? Why did it occur? What caused it? Does the child require further investigations or
treatment? Sometimes only a few questions reveal the problem; at
other times even detailed investigations fail to clarify the exact diagnosis. All this takes a great deal of experience on the part of the
physician who makes a diagnosis as if he or she were putting together a puzzle, piece by piece.

Many physicians and parents prefer to discuss the history alone
in order to have a freer exchange between them. It is very important
that children should also have this chance. They have their own feelings, worries, and little secrets, and they may find it difficult to share
them with the parents but not with the doctor. Physicians sometimes
interview the children separately from their parents but may all
come together at the end of the visit. Teenagers who talk more openly
when alone, are often seen first. Siblings should also be brought
along, introduced, and talked to so they don't feel excluded (see
Chapter 11).

Examination

The next step in the process of diagnosis is the physical and neurological examination. One can understand why a doctor stares into
eyes and ears, listens to the heart, and presses on tummies, but why
does he pound the knees with a little rubber hammer just to make the
legs jump? Why does he scratch the bottom of the foot and poke with
a sharp pin here and there? The neurological examination is often
mysterious or deceptively simple but it offers important information
regarding the various parts of the nervous system.

The doctor measures children's heads because when the size is
too small for their age, diminished brain growth is suspected;
this is often the case in brain damage. On the other hand, when the
head is larger than expected, long standing increased pressure inside the skull may be present (as in the case of hydrocephalus). Because the eye is an extension of the brain, its examination may offer
many clues in the diagnosis of neurological disorders.

Physicians carefully compare the sides of the body because
asymmetries are almost always abnormal. Scratching the outside of
the foot in normal children causes the toe to move down but when
one hemisphere is damaged the opposite toe may go up. Damage to
the right side of the brain could cause weakness and poor coordination of the left limbs and tapping the tendons over the joints may

produce overactive "deep tendon reflexes." Children with an abnormal cerebellum have poor coordination, unsteady gait, and a
tremor that is worse just before reaching an object. The doctor tests
these abilities by asking them to move their fingertip from the top of
their nose to the tip of his or her finger a short distance away.
Neurologists often state: "the examination showed hard (or soft)
neurological findings." "Hard" neurological signs mean obvious
abnormalities such as a markedly exaggerated deep tendon reflex,
weakness of a limb or a tremor. They are definite indicators of brain
damage. Clumsiness or slightly poor balance, on the other hand, are
less obvious and are examples of "soft" neurological signs. A careful
and expert neurological examination is of the greatest importance in
the investigation of a child with epilepsy and should be repeated at
regular intervals. Changes in the neurological findings may indicate the presence of drug toxicity, tumors, and progressive and other
brain disorders.

After history taking and examination, usually the physician
gives a preliminary impression and recommends further tests. The
doctor explains the information that contributed to this first impression and the reasons for the tests. It is inevitable that waiting for
these tests and for the results causes more anxiety. The physician is
aware of this hardship on the family and often is willing to phone the
parents or receive a call from them to communicate the results.

Brain Wave Test and the Preparation of the Child for It

The electroencephalogram (EEG) is one of the most important tests
for the investigation of epileptic disorders. It is always done during
the initial diagnostic period and repeated at regular intervals, as the
child is followed. Most people are aware of the importance of electrocardiogram in heart disease but they tend to be unaware of the existence of the EEG. The electrical activity of the brain can be recorded
in the same way as it is done for the heart (electrocardiogram) or
muscle (electromyogram). The test is entirely painless. It usually
lasts from 60 to 90 minutes. The technician carefully measures the
child's head and may make little colored marks with a pencil for
accurate placement of wires (electrodes) on the scalp. Through them
the electrical activity of the brain is picked up, magnified, and then
recorded by special pens on moving paper (Figure 1). The EEG is
continuously recorded when the children are awake, asleep, during
periods of deep breathing (if they are cooperative), and under special

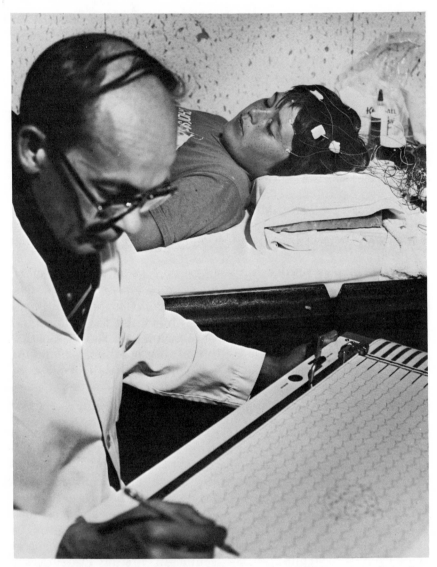

Figure 1.   The electrodes are pasted on carefully measured spots. There is no discomfort. The electrical activity of the brain is picked up, the current is magnified and then recorded by special pens on paper that moves from right to left.

types of bright, flickering light placed in front of their eyes. An EEG obtained only during wakefulness may be insufficient because drowsiness and sleep tend to bring out hidden abnormalities.

This recording, the EEG, frequently shows electrical disturbances in children with epilepsy. A seizure is a sudden, usually brief malfunction of the brain activity that may be compared to a sudden blurring of a television set. The interpretation of the electrical output of the brain, which changes continuously and looks chaotic to the unaccustomed eye, is a skill not easy to master. Abnormalities of this activity offer practical information about the underlying disorder. The EEG helps to identify the location, severity, cause, and type of seizure disorders. It may even help in formulating the prognosis (how well the seizures can be controlled) and in the selection of the most suitable anticonvulsant drugs. Certain special procedures are used routinely to further clarify the diagnosis. Prolonged deep breathing (hyperventilation) often precipitates absence seizures (petit mal) whereas exposure to flashing light (intermittent photic stimulation) activates typical electrical discharges in children with photosensitive epilepsy. Under special circumstances drugs may be injected intravenously to bring out hidden electrical abnormalities, or to suppress them. Occasionally wires are passed through the nostrils to the back of the throat (nasopharyngeal leads) to record electrical activity from the inner part of the temporal lobe. This is a delicate procedure because the nose and throat are sensitive but when the child is relaxed and cooperative it is not painful. A nasal decongestant or anesthetic spray may make the insertion of these electrodes easier. Very rarely it may be necessary to pass a long needle electrode through the cheeks in order to record seizure activity from the lowest part of the temporal lobe, which may not be detectable in regular EEG or nasopharyngeal recording. This is done under local anesthesia. Once the wires (sphenoidal electrodes) are inserted they can stay for days and nights, and multiple prolonged EEG recordings can be obtained.

The children should be prepared physically and emotionally for the EEG. Their hair should be washed thoroughly the day before so that the scalp is clean. They must know that the test does not hurt and their hair will not be shaved off. Most kids are scared of wires and may think that the EEG machine will give them shocks. They need to be reassured that this is not true. During the test they are thinking and relaxing, and their brain is generating energy like an electric battery. This goes through the wires and moves the pens. The result is a picture of how the brain works.

It is highly desirable that the children who are having a test see the EEG machine as a "magic box" rather than an instrument of torture. Indeed, this is what it may look like at first glance but electrodes glued to the head might be quite frightening. Although this will be clarified by the EEG technician who provides all sorts of reassurances, it is still likely that some of the children will feel unsafe at least for the first time. Thus, it is appropriate for the parents to spend some time with them discussing the various aspects of the test so that they know what to expect. They should be told that the EEG machine can not reveal what they are thinking. It may also be a good idea to make a drawing of the "magic box" that produces brain waves. Kids may enjoy being dressed up like an astronaut in a space craft imagining that the technician, who controls this mysterious machine, will take them for an adventurous trip. Children might be attracted by the many strange knobs and handles on the front panel. They can ask the technician to turn the lights and wheels on and off. They might be fascinated by the bright colors of the switchboard and may feel reassured if their favorite stuffed animal is allowed to have a couple of wires glued to its head. The EEG technicians who are used to dealing with kids know many ways to make them comfortable and how to decrease their apprehension. In exchange for their cooperation, at the end of the test the children may ask for a sample of the EEG. They could probably show this to relatives and friends.

Children may be requested to stay up for most of the preceding night in order to fall asleep naturally during the recording, on the following day. Usually they are delighted to be allowed, for once, to watch the "late show" on T.V. But for the parents it is not easy to entertain them for long hours. The following morning they likely will be tired and cranky. When the trip to the hospital is long it is important that they do not fall asleep in the car. If sleep deprivation has been unsuccessful the parents should inform the EEG technician upon arrival. If the children do not fall asleep on their own and if the doctor has not requested otherwise, there are harmless, liquid, short acting sedations that may be given. Young children love to have their favorite blanket and toy with them. Parents should not forget to bring them. For infants, the EEG may be arranged during nap times, with their bottles present. Some technicians allow the parents to stay during the test while others prefer them to wait outside, especially if the child is older. The technicians go through extensive training, which makes them knowledgeable about the abnormalities in the records. They cannot tell the parents or patients the results, however, because without knowing the whole medical history and other tests, the full meaning of the EEG is not clear. The technicians, though will ask parents about medications, type, severity, and frequency of the seizures. Such basic information is important to them in order to produce a meaningful and complete recording. Good technicians also know how to be helpful to patients irrespective of their age. Children need to be comfortable and relaxed so that their EEGs will be most informative for the doctor. While parents worry about the results, children want to be safe in that unfamiliar environment. They want to know that people will be friendly even if wearing white coats, that they will not be threatened or requested to do impossible things. If presented this way, the test may actually be an exciting and enjoyable experience.

Even when the seizures are well controlled, parents can expect that the EEGs will be periodically repeated. When the EEG shows more abnormalities than before, it is a warning to adjust the treatment. One of the basic rules of epilepsy is that without the permission of the physician, drugs should never be stopped abruptly. Anticonvulsants should not be discontinued prior to the EEG either. Unless specifically instructed otherwise, children should take their medications as usual. Occasionally though, under special diagnostic circumstances, physicians may gradually withdraw all drugs because they need to see seizure activity and the electrical abnormalities that are usually suppressed by the anticonvulsants. This is generally done in hospitals, however, where expert help is immediately available in case a child begins to have seizures excessively.

The Interpretation of EEGs

The EEG may be interpreted as normal or as showing specific or nonspecific abnormalities. A normal record means that it looks like that of most children at a particular age (Figure 2). The EEGs of children and especially of infants are more difficult to interpret because the range of normal variation is wider. A specific abnormality means that bursts of electrical activity never seen in normal conditions have been recorded over certain areas of the brain. The correlation of a specific EEG abnormality with the detailed description of the seizures leads to the diagnosis of a particular form of epilepsy. At times a seizure may occur during the EEG (Figure 3). The presence of electrical abnormalities ("discharges") accompanying seizure activity prove beyond dispute the epileptic nature of the condition. This does not happen very often, however, especially when the child is

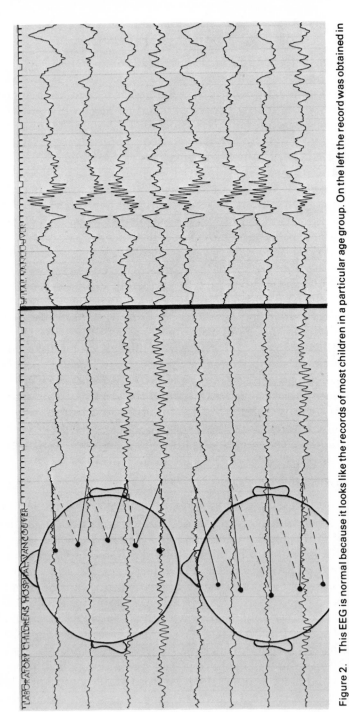

Figure 2.   This EEG is normal because it looks like the records of most children in a particular age group. On the left the record was obtained in wakefulness while on the right during sleep.

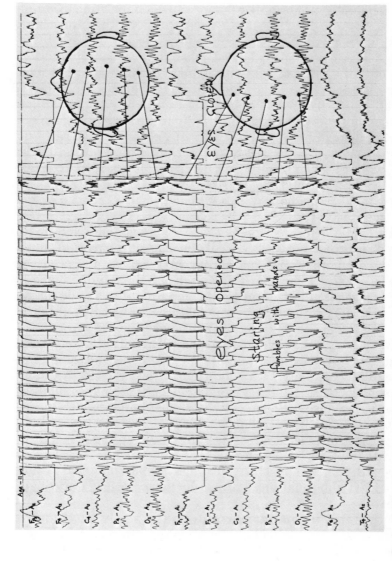

Figure 3. During this small segment of EEG recording the child had a seizure. Note the bursts of electrical discharges as they stand out from the ongoing background. This paroxysmal activity is accompanied by momentary loss of consciousness. The child was diagnosed as having absence seizures (petit mal).

under treatment and the seizures are rare. Therefore, the neurologist has to rely on discrete but specific EEG discharges that may be recorded although the child does not exhibit evidence of a seizure.

A nonspecific abnormality is more difficult to define in simple words. It refers to patterns of brain wave activity that are usually seen in children with neurological problems, such as hyperactivity, learning disabilities, delayed development or poor coordination. In other words, the EEGs of a sizeable number of children without convulsive disorders have such findings. This includes a number of "normal" children as well. For instance those who have had simple febrile convulsions (see Chapter 6) without further evidence of epilepsy may also exhibit, especially at a certain age, unusual patterns. They may appear in the EEG only during certain states, for instance, while the child is falling asleep. They may be seen in certain areas of the brain, usually on both sides or all over, and all at once. In this case the neurologist states that the EEG shows some paroxysmal activity.

Paroxysmal refers to a burst of activity that stands out from the ongoing background of the EEG. All abnormal discharges of epileptic nature are paroxysmal, but paroxysmal activity also occurs in physiological states such as during sleep of normal individuals.

The presence of these nonspecific abnormalities should not necessarily be alarming because such features in the EEG, although properly described as abnormal, do not make the diagnosis of epilepsy. What counts is the degree and persistence of such nonspecific findings and how they correlate with the symptoms and complaints of the child. They may be an indicator of low seizure threshold, which means greater tendency (compared to the normal population) to have a convulsion under certain predisposing circumstances. When the situation is such that the threat of a seizure is very high, the physician may elect to treat as if the child had epilepsy. For example, in Chapter 6, a young girl with an atypical febrile convulsion is discussed. Her benign seizure disorder was accompanied by nonspecific EEG abnormalities and her doctor prescribed anticonvulsant therapy.

Finally, it is important to realize that a small percentage of youngsters with true epileptic seizures may show no discharges or just nonspecific EEG findings. Parents should realize that the chance of detecting a latent EEG abnormality is proportional to the completeness of the study (length of recording in both waking and sleeping, use of special electrodes, procedures, and so on). Thus, if the

EEG is normal at the first attempt, it may have to be repeated shortly with the appropriate arrangements or in a different laboratory.

X-rays and the CAT Scan

During the investigation of epilepsy, frequently a skull x-ray is ordered. Skull x-rays are usually normal because only the bone and not the brain shows up. The doctor wants to make sure there are no deposits of calcium in the brain, bony deformities, or asymmetries that may suggest the presence of a tumor (Figure 4). A more useful and informative new test is the CAT scan (computerized axial tomog-

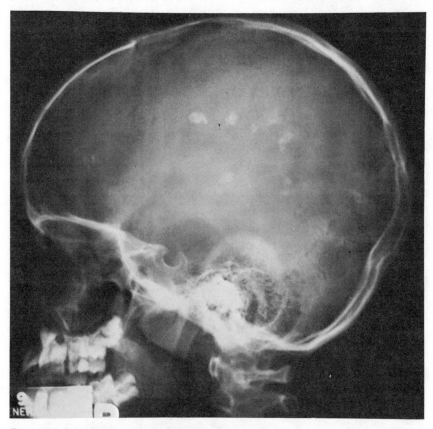

Figure 4.   This skull x-ray reveals several small areas of calcifications. The child has tuberous sclerosis—a hereditary brain disorder. The cause of seizures is easily explained.

raphy). This painless procedure is performed as the child lies comfortably on his or her back while a series of x-ray probes disposed all around the head send in beams each from a different angle. A computer, measuring the amount of x-ray absorbed in each single point of the brain, pieces the images together and a picture of a section of the head appears on a TV screen (Figure 5, Figure 6). Thanks to this remarkable machine the physician can now carefully examine the brain. Although this test is constantly being improved so that images are clearer and more detailed, tiny abnormalities may not be seen.

Most laboratories give clear instructions to the parents before the CAT scan is done. Parents should prepare their children because they are easily frightened by large machines, busy doctors, and technicians dressed in white coats and conversing in a strange technical language. They may be upset by the sight of a sick patient in a wheelchair or on a stretcher. There may be the smell of hospital wards. Much of this unnecessary anxiety can be eliminated with appropriate information and reassurance.

The CAT scan usually lasts from 30 to 45 minutes. Occasionally a special dye is injected into the blood stream in order to get a better

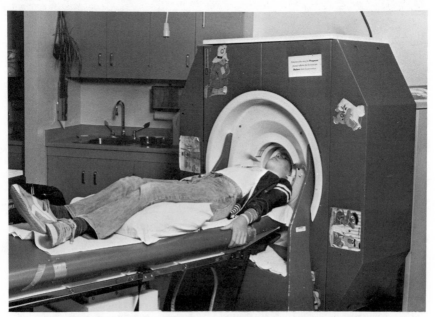

Figure 5.   The child lies comfortably while the CAT scan is being done.

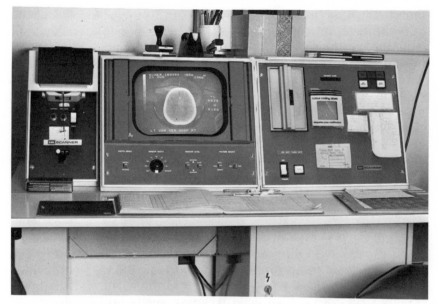

Figure 6.   The computer creates the image of the brain in sections.

view of the affected structures of the brain. Although most technicians are skillful in dealing with children, parents might wish to
remain with the child. This might be possible but it is not encouraged
because of the unnecessary exposure to even minute amounts of radiation. The child must lie quietly because movements blur the images, making this important test quite useless. Therefore, children
who do not cooperate or are not able to hold their heads absolutely
still for a few minutes at a time require sedation or a brief period of
anesthesia. Solid foods and milk should be avoided for at least 3
hours before the examination because sedation may cause nausea. If
groggy children vomit, it may get aspirated into their lungs, causing
pneumonia. Water, gingerale, and even jello, however, can safely be
given. The images of the brain are developed immediately after the
test and the neuroradiologist, another specialist in the teamwork,
carefully studies them and sends a report to the referring physician.

Blood Tests

Investigations of epilepsy always include blood tests. The physician
needs to know about the blood sugar, calcium, biochemical abnormalities, or whether infection is present. Functions of various or-

gans in the body (liver and kidneys especially) must be tested in view of possible treatment with drugs. Whenever possible, it should be explained to the child how and when blood is taken. The parents must never say it does not hurt because it does and then the child can become more frightened or distrustful. Usually a single sample is enough for all the tests. Blood is sometimes taken from the finger but usually from the arm after a tourniquet is put on and the area is cleansed with alcohol. The pain resembles a mosquito bite and is quickly over. We have all been children, however, and have not forgotten how frightening is the anticipation of the needle! It is wise to praise them afterward for being so brave. Most of them are.

Spinal Tap

A spinal tap is not required frequently; when it is, it should be done when the child is admitted to a hospital. (See Febrile seizures in Chapter 6.) The brain produces fluid (cerebro-spinal fluid), which circulates from the cerebral ventricles to the surface of the brain (Figure 2, Chapter 2). Like blood, it contains cells, protein, sugar, and other biochemical substances, and thus it helps the physician make a diagnosis.

During the spinal tap the child sits on the bed or lies on his or her side. The lower part of the spine is carefully cleaned with disinfectant, and the area of the puncture is infiltrated with a local anesthetic in order to avoid pain. Then a special needle is passed between two vertebrae into the spinal canal and some fluid is drained off. To avoid leakage at the puncture site, the child should stay still in bed for at least 30 minutes and lie quietly for the rest of the day. The more relaxed the child is, the easier it is to do this test. This procedure does not cause low back pain in later life, as some believe. Sometimes after a spinal tap, a child may complain of a headache for a few hours but it is a harmless test, and in the hands of experts it is nearly painless.

Pneumoencephalogram and Angiogram

The treating physician after hearing the opinion of other specialists may come to the conclusion that a *pneumoencephalogram* or *angiogram* is necessary. These tests require general anesthesia and therefore, hospitalization. Parents need to feel comfortable with this decision and should ask their physicians to explain what additional information they hope to obtain and why it might be useful.

The pneumoencephalogram (air bubble test) is done under a general anesthetic. Through a spinal tap, some cerebro-spinal fluid is removed and replaced with equal amounts of air. Because air is lighter than the fluid, the bubbles travel up to the cavities of the brain (ventricles). When x-rays of the skull are taken, the ventricles filled with air show up as black shadows. Physicians can then study their shape very carefully, looking for any distortion. The bubbles soon disappear because the gas is gradually dissolved and reabsorbed into the blood stream, but most children will complain bitterly of headaches for 1 or 2 days. They feel miserable and may even vomit shortly after the test. The advent of CAT scans has reduced greatly the need for this investigation. In certain cases, however, it provides invaluable clues for the definite diagnosis.

The angiograms are done by injecting a dye into one of the arteries leading to the brain. X-rays are taken moments after the injection and the arteries show up like a snow covered tree on a winter night. Again the brain can be studied by knowing how arteries usually appear; in addition, any abnormality affecting the blood vessels can be detected. Parents should have no reservations about asking for an explanation of these tests beforehand.

Hospitalization

While it is desirable to prevent hospitalization of children, with epilepsy it is not always possible to do so; sometimes it is necessary. Unfortunately, they are frequently admitted without preparation due to the emergency nature of their disorder.

Preschoolers are not accustomed to meeting people such as the house staff, nurses, cleaning persons, technicians, or orderlies. Separation from their families makes it hard for them to cope. Many believe their admission to hospital is a punishment for something they have done. Their anxieties can be reduced by preparing them so that their overall experiences are positive, not negative. When possible it is advisable for the parents and children to visit the hospital in advance as well as the unit to which they will be admitted. This one-to-one preparation is the most effective.

If parents know that their young children will be hospitalized, a good book to read with them is *"Curious George Goes to the Hospital"* (Rey and Rey, 1966). This story describes many aspects of hospital life in a funny, lighthearted way. Also, *"A Trip to the Hospital"* book can be written. It should include what they can expect, where parents will be, the usual ward routines and visiting schedules. An older child could read Weber's *"Elizabeth Gets Well"* (Weber, 1969) and *"My Friend The Doctor"* (Watson, Switzer, and Hirschberg, 1972).

Children need to be given an opportunity to understand and discuss their worries about being hospitalized. Parents, of course, should listen. Misconceptions can be formed from incomplete fragments of information. Parents must tell the truth and should not try to change their children's feelings. If a child is anxious, it is better to say, "I know it is scary but this or that can help" rather than "Don't be scared." Children are excellent detectors of emotions. Therefore, parents also need to express their feelings; for example, "Yes, dad is sad about your going to the hospital but our doctor tells us it's best for you." Parents should tell their children that they expect them to go along with the hospital rules even though it may be hard.

Role playing can be used even after the preschool age. Children are asked to pretend that the parents are the children and then to treat them as "patients" just as they expect it is in a hospital. There could be a lot of mean treatment! Acknowledging these hardships is one way of letting the children know that the parents do understand. These frustrations can remind all of us that we still have much to learn and do. All explanations need to be given several times. After the first discussion, a little time should be allowed to pass. Then the children are asked to explain the situation so that the parents can recognize some of their feelings or worries. Again the discussion is repeated. It can also be mentioned that although the children have the hardest job, they, the parents, and the doctors are all working together. Of course, a balance is needed in such an approach. It is fine to expect children to be "big" but their fears, anger, and sadness must also be expressed. These feelings are always easier to tolerate when they are brought into the open and discussed.

As the child and the parent enter the hospital, admission papers are filled out. An identification bracelet is given, which is generally worn on the wrist. Then they are taken to the ward where the investigations and treatment are to be carried out. The nurses usually get an idea from the parents about the daily routine, likes and dislikes, and they introduce other children by their first names. Although the family physician or the specialist already knows the child well, invariably another history and examination are obtained by one, and often two of the house staff. Repeating the same history so many times may seem senseless to parents who already are fatigued by the emotional and complicated procedures of the hospitalization. But afterward, doctors, nurses, and other hospital personnel involved will compare notes for a better understanding of the case, for better care and treatment. Following this, orders are written on the hospital chart for investigations and treatment. All this looks frightening to a young child and restrictive to an adolescent. Children (like most of us) can manage unpleasant experiences a little better when able to make some of their own choices. For instance, it is helpful to allow them to pick the arm from which blood is to be taken or if they wish, to have the hospital bracelet put on either before or after a certain procedure.

Parents can make the hospital admission a more pleasant and positive experience for the child. They should bring in clothes, familiar favorite toys and books with the child's name on them. Toys, books, and magazines can reduce the strangeness of the environment, attract other children, and make the separation of the family less traumatic as well as make the waiting seem not so long. Older children should bring their school books so that they can study with hospital teachers.

Today pediatric hospitals have very liberal rules for the visiting members of the family. There are regular and often unrestricted visiting hours for parents throughout the day. It is difficult to believe that 30–40 years ago families were limited to one brief visit a week. Parents should spend as much time as possible with their young children. Not infrequently, parents hesitate and even avoid visiting because the youngsters are upset after they leave. This is clearly wrong. Children must not be allowed to feel deserted. The occasional phone call, get well card from members of the family and friends, bringing a brother or sister to visit or perhaps a new toy make the hospitalized child feel that he or she is still very much part of the family. Although young children do not have good time concept, it is surprising how many of them watch the clock prior to visiting hours, so parents should not be late in arriving.

Many hospitals provide school programs and well organized play activities. For the older child, going to school is a normal activity and as such helps to reduce the strangeness of a hospital. For the younger child, play is not a frivolous matter but a necessity. Recognizing the needs of preschoolers, some hospitals have units where the parents can also live, and for teenagers, some provide adolescent wards with appropriate recreational activities.

After discharge, younger children who have been accompanied to the hospital by their parents and have kept close contact with the family, make the transition from hospital to home without much emotional upheaval. At the other extreme, children may exhibit various patterns of adverse behavior on arriving home but this generally resolves itself in a few days or weeks. If there seems to be a persistent problem, it should be mentioned to the doctor. He or she may have some useful advice or ask someone else to help.

References and Suggested Reading

Rey, H. A., and Rey, M. 1966. Curious George Goes to The Hospital. Houghton, Mifflin Company, Boston.
Watson, J. W., Switzer, R. E., and Hirschberg, J. C. 1972. My Friend The Doctor. Golden Press, New York.
Weber, A. 1969. Elizabeth Gets Well. Thomas Crowell Co., New York.

chapter 4

Primary (Idiopathic) Generalized Epilepsy

Absence Seizures (Petit Mal)
Convulsive Seizures (Grand Mal)
Light-Sensitive Seizures
Suggested Reading

Depending on which part of the brain is involved in the electrical disturbance, seizures vary in their appearance (Figure 1). The earliest classification of these patterns was aimed at differentiating real seizures from hysterical ones (seizures related to psychogenic causes). Thus grand mal, petit mal, and hysteroid types were introduced, but such oversimplification turned out to be unsatisfactory. Over the years innumerable terms emerged to describe certain types of seizures, again leading to confusion. Because uniformity was crucial for international scientific communication, the Commission on Classification of the International League Against Epilepsy has been developing a more useful classification since 1969.

This system is based on the fact that some seizures from the beginning involve the entire brain at once, called primary (idiopathic) generalized while others are focal (partial) first and then may or may not become secondarily generalized.

The primary (idiopathic) generalized seizures can be further divided into nonconvulsive and convulsive attacks. The best example of the first type is an absence seizure (petit mal) and of the second is grand mal, also known as a tonic-clonic seizure. Both are common. Most of these children have normal intelligence and are average or above average students despite their medical problem. They are not predisposed to having additional handicaps and lack any evidence of brain damage. These forms of epilepsy are often inherited (see Chapter 11). When abnormalities are present in the EEG (spike and wave discharges), they are always over both hemispheres. Otherwise, as the children grow, the maturation of their EEG patterns is normal.

Absence Seizures (Petit Mal)

Seven-year-old Mary Westmore lives in a charming little town. She was well until the age of 4 when her parents became aware of blinking episodes during which she vacantly stared into space for 5 to 10 seconds. These would intrude on her conversation, playing, eating, or other ac-

THE ORIGIN of SYMPTOMS and SIGNS in FOCAL SEIZURES

A visual display over the dominant hemisphere

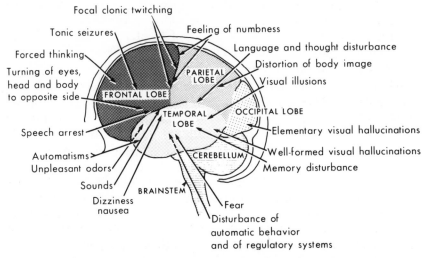

Figure 1.   The origin of symptoms and signs in focal seizures.

tivities. At first her parents were annoyed—they thought Mary had picked up a bad habit. They asked her to stop it and this confused and upset Mary who did not seem to hear or see during these spells nor had she any memory of the events. When the blinking episodes were over she would try to continue her interrupted activity or even pick up the conversation where she had left off. The parents did not discuss this problem with their pediatrician for over a year.

During an annual check-up, the parents mentioned the problem to the pediatrician who strongly suspected absence seizures (petit mal). He arranged for an EEG in the nearest city where the diagnosis was confirmed and the treatment was started. Although there were fewer attacks, the medications failed to stop them entirely. Drugs were added and discontinued but the absence seizures were never fully controlled.

In kindergarten, Mary was described by her teachers as a sleepy, tired, and inattentive girl. She was passed into the first grade because she was considered to be smart; her academic progress, however, proved to be so slow that the school recommended special class attendance. The parents found this very upsetting. During this period they took Mary to several physicians.

Finally, Mr. and Mrs. Westmore were referred to a seizure clinic for a comprehensive assessment. A new anticonvulsant drug was started. Within a week Mary's staring spells disappeared and her EEG improved. Slowly, the other drugs were discontinued. Mary became a bright, talkative, and charming little girl. She no longer had trouble with her school work.

Literally, petit mal means a "small seizure" but in medical terminology it represents a specific disorder with characteristic EEG pattern. Suddenly the consciousness is interrupted for from 5 to 15 seconds without any drowsiness afterward. These children may have a few or several hundred spells a day and in these cases their learning can be severely affected (see Chapter 13). The EEG typically shows sudden bursts of 3 spike and waves per second simultaneously over both hemispheres. These electrical abnormalities are usually precipitated by prolonged deep breathing (Figure 6, Chapter 3). If the generalized discharge lasts longer than 3 to 5 seconds, absence seizures become apparent. The pattern may differ. Those who have pure petit mal simply stare ahead. Rhythmic blinking or twitching of the mouth and arms in exact synchrony with the electrical discharges occur in some.

When the spell is prolonged some individuals may carry out stereotyped motor movements (automatisms) like twiddling with their clothes or tapping on furniture but they are completely unaware of doing this. Such automatisms may also be seen in other types of epilepsy. It is important to differentiate absence seizures from other types of staring spells such as those seen in certain types of complex partial seizures (as temporal lobe epilepsy) because the medical treatment is entirely different.

During these absence spells the electrical storms of spike and wave discharges seem to involve the entire cortex but have little influence on functions controlled by areas of the brain below. This is why children, during their petit mal attacks, are completely unaware of their environment but do not collapse.

Absence seizures usually begin during the second half of the first decade and may disappear by puberty although the onset could be earlier or later. Rarely do they continue into adulthood. The majority of affected children are normal in every other aspect.

Zarontin is the most commonly used drug. Generalized convulsions sometimes occur with absence seizures. Depakene, a recently introduced anticonvulsant, is especially useful and will control both petit mal and convulsions. There are still other less commonly used drugs (see Chapter 8).

Ann Walker, a 12-year-old, with well controlled petit mal was on Zarontin and Diamox for several months. One week she became excessively lethargic. Her teacher called home from school because Ann appeared to be distant and continuously had to be reminded what to do. The teacher felt that perhaps the medications were "too strong" for the girl. The next day the father took Ann to her neurologist who immediately ordered an EEG. After reviewing the test, the physician explained that

she was having petit mal status (continuous seizures). The EEG
showed continuous irregular spike and wave discharges in contrast to
the previous record, which was almost normal. The constant abnormal
electrical activity interfered with her thinking and this was why Ann
looked so stunned. She was not taking too much medication but rather
too little. The physician added that sometimes after several months Diamox loses its anticonvulsant effect. Although Ann's seizures were well
controlled before, she outgrew the doses of her medications and this
allowed the petit mal to appear in full force in status.

Ann was hospitalized and then was given intravenous Valium,
which seemed to snap her out of her lethargy. The doses of Zarontin and
Diamox were also increased. The next day she was feeling normal
again.

Petit mal status is rare. It occurs more commonly in adults who
had idiopathic generalized epilepsy in their childhood. The seizure
disorder is often confused with a schizophrenic breakdown because
these individuals are distant and may seem strange.

Absence seizures (petit mal) usually appear after the parents
have been able to manage most of the trials and tribulations of early
childhood—sleep-disrupting cries, mollifying paces across the bed-
room floor, recurrent small crises of illnesses and falls, the preschooler's crayon experiments on the living room wall. They had
endured these experiences and more. They have come to know the
personality and temperament of their children. Now, epilepsy, "The
intruder," enters the life and routine of the young family.

At first, the parents may observe only a slight change in the
child. For the child, it is scarcely noticeable. After all, these are just
moments of blinking, staring, or an interruption in an activity. In
perhaps half of the youngsters (as in other types of seizures), however, there are also associated behavioral difficulties. These are irritability, tiredness, less spontaneity, increased activity level, and
some problems in the parent-child relationship. With appropriate
medical treatment, in over 50% of these children most of the changes
disappear. For those who continue to have problems, a better understanding of good child management practices and developmental
stages will allow compensatory changes in the family.

An acute and chronic disorder, epilepsy subjects the child and
the parents to recurrent, unexpected attacks with unpredictable frequency. It affects their sense of control, and when that is continually
disrupted, the family must find some way of dealing with the predicament. The parents may either constantly over-restrain the child or
take no control at all. Both are extremes. Acceptance, patience, and
understanding, however, can help in this situation.

Normal Reactions

Once epilepsy is diagnosed the parents usually ask certain questions. "Why did this happen to us? How can we manage our family now? What kind of activities are reasonable for us?" The type of answers will provide the base of a successful adaptation or will result in further complications.

Why? At best the answer will permit the family to accept the unknown and deal with the anxieties of a difficult situation. At worst, it can lead to increasing blame and guilt, which will interfere with the medical treatment and may create dismay in the family unit.

How? At best, the parents approach each problem with a number of well thought out ideas. Blanket denial (nothing is wrong!) is the worst approach because the family then ignores that something is different and troublesome. Such denial not only interferes with parental responsibility but it may eventually influence the child to refuse medications or to enter life-endangering situations.

What? Even people with difficult illnesses can learn to manage their lives. Children and their families need to be involved in stimulating, relationship-maintaining, and growth-producing activities. Avoidance, defensive restriction, over-activity, or careless disregard do not foster development. The family rules must be clear; concerns should be discussed and clarified.

Ways a Child May Be Affected

The parents' answers will exert a powerful influence on the child who also thinks about the same questions. If the family decides that a particular person or event is responsible for the epilepsy, not only can a relationship be disrupted for the child but the blame may interfere with the acceptance of the seizures. Alternatively, if the child is blamed for the pain and inconvenience, a sense of guilt in all concerned may result. When the parents decide to ignore a problem totally or find themselves consumed by it, the child may do the same. How and what parents will allow will strongly influence what the child believes is possible.

Autonomy and competence are important aspects of the development of children. Autonomy refers to the degree of control people feel over themselves and their lives. Competence is defined as the degree of ability individuals experience with tasks in the physical environment. As a result of a brief electrical discharge, epilepsy ruptures the personal power over one's sense of self and over one's body. It can entangle interpersonal relationships and force others to assume responsibility. This, in turn, can exert a major effect on the evolution of the children's sense of competence. Because seizures represent an actual disruption of control, the family may be less willing to grant them autonomy. This curtailment of freedom, in turn, reduces the number of situations in which these children can act and to that extent decreases opportunities for learning. Epilepsy may also have a direct impact on their sense of competence since "to be ill is to do poorly." Additionally, the learning disorders that occasionally may be present diminish their ability to solve problems and to be competent—yet another factor in making the family reluctant to grant autonomy.

Medications and Feelings

While medication is a valuable aid in the treatment of epilepsy, the sense of self-control is quite different. Anticonvulsants may or may not stop the seizures. This presents different problems for each child throughout development.

In the relative absence of seizures, the rare, isolated attack can have frightening consequences for the children. Medication can either be a reminder of their lack of self-control or of a sense of dependence. This can make them feel angry or sad. In either case their subjective sense of control or autonomy may be affected, and these natural feelings should be discussed.

Children who achieve intermediate control must consolidate some stable defense mechanisms to cope with the occasional seizure. They should "think about the good things," "live day by day," or think they are "learning something special" through this problem but they also need to acknowledge that sometimes they feel angry or scared or sad (the usual emotions). Their defense mechanisms (and their relationship to the family's) can appear in a striking fashion in young adulthood. The youngster, who prior to and during early adolescence may have done well by disregarding the seizures can now become much more resistant to accepting responsibility for taking medication or became more apathetic about other responsibilities. The disregard has turned into disbelief.

In those with very poor control the seizures are a more constant issue. Because of the continuous state of anxiety to which the child and the family are exposed, the slow progress toward consolidation of autonomy and self-control is more painfully evident. The attitudes of the parents and their ability to support (or overprotect) the child are also highlighted.

Thus, although drugs may prevent seizures, the feelings of children are still affected. In order to "control" their lives they remain painfully aware of their dependence on medications.

What to Tell a Child?

Children are capable of taking many medical disorders in their stride and can adapt ingeniously. During this process of adaptation, with proper support and acknowledgment of their feelings, they can develop their own positive attitudes in accepting the problems. This acceptance can be supported by providing clear information that children can understand and by clarifying their emotions in a non-judgmental way.

Helping children handle information is a step by step process. For example, if the parents know that the child is coming to the hospital for a test, it is possible to plan a trip beforehand. The family can explore the hospital together so that the child can discover that it is a place that promotes health and where sick people get better. During the visit the parents should mention that they will come again. If the children are interested they will ask more questions. If not, a little later in the week, one can review the last trip and give more information about what will be done to them. Extra questions may also be asked during the week. Many parents find this type of communication difficult because they do not wish to worry their child. While talking about a hospital trip may lead to some worry, anger, or sadness, these feelings should be acknowledged as natural. The end result is that these children will be more comfortable than if things are sprung on them at the last minute or if they begin to react to the tension of secret planning in the household about an unannounced trip.

Children, by the age of 3 or 4, can understand that the brain sends messages to different parts of the body, just like the heart circulates blood or when someone makes telephone calls. One can tell them that sometimes there is a little extra electricity in one part of the brain, which leads to these attacks. (The nature of the seizure is described. It can even be imitated.) It can be stated that this is just like people talking or walking in their sleep. The brain is sending out a message that a person did not willingly initiate. The same is true of a seizure—the extra electricity in one part of the brain sends out an unwanted message. If the child says "that's ickky" or "I don't want to listen," parents can sympathize by saying something that reflects their understanding such as, "yes, that can make you mad" or "sad things are hard to listen to." When it seems difficult to continue a discussion it should be left alone for a while or until the child brings it up or a parent can try again during a comfortable moment. The medications can be explained as something that prevents the brain from sending out those unwanted messages.

Each visit to the doctor can be an opportunity to increase information about epilepsy. For many children and families, once the seizures are well controlled and the initial phase of acceptance has been accomplished, the main message to be conveyed is that the medicine is a good helper. This fosters the acceptance of the medication routine as part of their life so that later, taking anticonvulsants regularly does not become a problem. Even then the child may occasionally refer to feeling angry about going to the doctor or about having to remember the pills. It is worthwhile to continue to ask about those feelings and to acknowledge them as long as they will not be an "excuse" for unacceptable behavior.

Convulsive Seizures (Grand Mal)

Ten-year-old Chris Stonner was the daughter of a dentist. She and her younger sister were healthy all their lives and did well in school. During a Christmas vacation, the family flew to Disneyland for their first visit and it was, indeed, an exciting time for them all. On their second day there in the late afternoon, Chris suddenly let out a short muffled cry and fell to the floor of the hotel lobby. For 10 to 20 seconds her body was stiff and trembling and she did not breathe. Then rhythmically her arms and legs began to jerk so violently that at one point her body was thrown right around. After a minute or so, the jerking stopped and Chris fell into a deep sleep.

Neither Dr. Stonner nor his wife had ever seen a seizure before although they recognized it as such. As a dentist, Dr. Stonner knew not to put any hard object between his daughter's teeth because of the danger of harming them and all he did was to protect her from injury. People gathered around the child and the hotel clerk called for the nurse on duty. It was hard for the family when people began making "helpful" suggestions such as, "Hold her tongue, she will swallow it!" "Give her oxygen or she will suffocate!" One of the tourists shouted for an ambulance. Mrs. Stonner, who had never in her life been so frightened, overheard a mother explaining to her children that "the poor little girl is an epileptic."

The nurse was there within a couple of minutes, picked up the child, who had wet herself during the convulsion, and took her to the First Aid

Station. The frightened Mrs. Stonner kept asking her, "Is she going to die?" Ten minutes later Chris was awake, wondering what had happened. When the ambulance arrived the family was taken to the emergency ward of the nearest hospital where the diagnosis of a seizure was made. The Christmas vacation ended with one blow—Chris had become an "epileptic."

Later, Chris had detailed neurological investigations. All were normal except for the brain wave test. She began taking phenobarbital tablets; her medical diagnosis was idiopathic generalized epilepsy (grand mal). Her progress in school continued to be good and she remained seizure free.

During a primary generalized convulsive seizure (grand mal) the electric discharges instantaneously involve the entire brain, therefore, there is no warning. Consciousness is lost from the beginning. Some individuals are irritable and restless before an attack. In contrast, focal seizures may become generalized later in which case there is often an initial warning (aura) before the loss of consciousness. Children with grand mal suddenly become stiff (tonic phase) and unconscious, fall to the ground and may bite their tongue. There is often a strange cry because as the muscles of the chest contract the air rushes out between the vocal cords, making a sound. This does not indicate pain. Because of increased pressure in the bladder and bowel there may be wetting (urinary incontinence) or soiling (fecal incontinence). Then the extremities begin to jerk rhythmically (clonic phase). The saliva that is not swallowed during the attack appears as frothing at the mouth. Because the muscles of respiration are also involved, breathing is irregular. The seizure is usually over within a few minutes but a deep sleep for up to several hours follows.

A post-ictal state (after the attack) is to be expected after a major grand mal convulsion. During this period it may be difficult to wake the child or even to obtain any kind of response. The reflexes are depressed or abnormal. That is why this state is also referred to as post-ictal coma. Many parents who have not seen generalized convulsions before often erroneously think that the children are unconscious because of a head injury they may have sustained during the fall or even that they are dying. Thus, after the shocking experience of witnessing a grand mal seizure, the post-ictal state may also be terrifying. The breathing can be so shallow that the parents fear a respiratory arrest (the cessation of normal respiration). Actually if parents could overcome their overwhelming apprehension, it is apparent that these children are breathing peacefully. The normal color of the skin should reassure the parents that the child is getting enough oxygen. The post-ictal state is probably due to exhaustion of the brain cells and it may represent a useful stage for recharging energy. Therefore, excessive stimulation is unwise. The storm is over. The child is exhausted but safe and should rest.

After waking up, the tired child may have a throbbing headache for which an analgesic could be given. There is no recollection of the events. During the seizure there is no pain although this is a common worry for the parents. Injury may occur during the fall, or, the clonic period. Children with epilepsy cannot swallow their tongues although they may bite them. The management of a person during a seizure is discussed in Chapter 9.

It is not unusual for the first convulsion to occur in later childhood; this is puzzling to the parents who frequently ask: "If my child has epilepsy, why didn't it show up just after birth?" As discussed in Chapter 2, different seizure disorders have different ages of onset (Chapter 2, Figure 5). Primary generalized convulsions, which are often hereditary, can surface even during the second or third decades of life, although they may be preceded by petit mal or myoclonic jerks.

The majority of these children have no evidence of brain damage and do well in life. By and large, the later the onset in childhood, the better the outlook for seizure control. Treatment is generally successful with a number of anticonvulsants, sometimes in combination, such as, barbiturates (phenobarbital, Mysoline, and Mebaral), Dilantin, Tegretol, and Depakene. Although the duration of therapy is debatable, many physicians gradually discontinue the medication after a long seizure-free period (see Chapter 7). For good control of epilepsy, extreme tiredness should be avoided, therefore, the child's lifestyle and sleeping habits should be regular. Chris's first seizure may have been precipitated by her overtiredness.

The Management of Fear

Absence seizures (petit mal) are in many ways the most easily tolerated. The attacks are brief and involve little physical change. They are usually easily controlled and there is hope that with time the spells will be "outgrown." While primary generalized convulsions (grand mal) may also disappear, although less frequently, the attacks last longer and are more dramatic. Fortunately, they also tend to respond to treatment. Anticipating a major convulsion (grand mal), however, is more troublesome than tolerating an occasional staring spell. The dramatic nature of these attacks increases the problems associated with psychological reactions for both parents and child.

As discussed above, it is natural to ask "Why me? How can I stand this? What can I do?" It is also normal for a child to feel angry about "being stuck with this thing" and to wish for it to go away or belong to someone else. It is natural for parents to feel worried, frightened, disappointed, angry, sad, and sometimes guilty. When the feelings begin to control the individual rather than vice versa, however, there is a new problem to solve. Fear is the most troublesome in relation to generalized convulsions. It is natural because there are dangers. Anxieties and tensions are easily communicated (even nonverbally) so that the reaction of one member of the family can heighten that of others. All of these make it hard to sort out how to manage our fears about major convulsions. If the anxiety of the family is transmitted to children, their fears may interfere with activities or feelings about themselves. The most troublesome outcome is when children feel manipulated by the emotional reactions of the family. For example, if the parents' fears lead to a variety of prohibitions, the children may be angry about being deprived of certain activities and may decide to try to manipulate the reaction of the family in order to get their way. Awareness of this can help avoid this kind of problem; the situation can then be discussed rather than everyone just acting on their feelings.

The Management of Uncertainty

Uncertainty, which is just as troublesome as fear, is part of having seizures. The fact that so often the reason for epilepsy is unclear and that frequently all the investigations are normal can foster this feeling. Realizing that a cause might be found (relief) but that it might be a tumor (fear) is a double-edged sword. It is hard not knowing why a child has seizures; it is more difficult to think that a cause that lurks inside the body or the brain may be discovered later.

Fluctuations in seizure control, the delay or lack of response to initial therapy, the possibility of developing side-effects from medications, and other doubtful feelings must be dealt with. The partnership between the family and the physician should create some comfort because the doctor's knowledge and guidance can help the parents and the child bear these uncertainties. Besides, such alliance will generate an atmosphere of awareness and cooperation about finding out what is best for the child according to the circumstances. Having a more active role in this process makes uncertainty more acceptable.

Light-Sensitive Seizures

For 3 years Ed Clark, a 15-year-old healthy teenager, had occasional involuntary jerks of his arms especially in the morning when getting ready for school. He did not mention this to anyone because he thought it was just nervousness. Once in history class he was carefully drawing a map when he suddenly involuntarily scribbled over the drawing. Ed felt frustrated. Another time, on a Sunday morning, after spilling some orange juice, his mother reprimanded him for being careless; he was hurt because he had been careful. The same day the family took a long car ride to the beach. On the way back Ed dozed off in the rear seat when the sunlight shining through the trees began to flicker on his face. Suddenly his whole body stiffened up and he started to shake violently.

Ed woke up in the hospital emergency room where the nurse informed him that he had had a convulsion. "Don't worry, it is all over now. You are perfectly alright." The doctors found out that an uncle of Ed's was still being treated for grand mal epilepsy. They asked if he had ever had any blackout spells before and Ed suddenly remembered about those jerking episodes. The physicians felt that those were probably brief myoclonic seizures that sometimes precede major convulsions.

The neurological examination was normal. The explanation as to why he convulsed came from the EEG which was done a couple of days later (Figure 2). The tracing was normal in all respects except during intermittent photic stimulation, when the light placed in front of his eyes flickered 10 times per second or more, and big electrical discharges were generated by his brain. During this test once or twice he felt his muscles twitch just like before but the EEG technician was careful to expose him to the flickering lights only for short periods of time. The doctor explained that if these periods were longer major convulsions could develop; nevertheless, the test showed that Ed had a form of hereditary seizure disorder called *light-sensitive epilepsy*. He went on telling that Ed's convulsion was triggered by the rapid alternation of bright sunshine and shadows while they were driving past the trees. In this type of photoconvulsive epilepsy, uncontrollable spontaneous myoclonic jerks may also occur, frequently shortly after getting up in the morning or on sudden exposure to bright light. Such individuals may be so sensitive that simple eye opening or closing could cause electrical discharges in the EEG. Their predisposition to this type of light sensitivity is inherited. Otherwise, this is a benign, well-tolerated form of epilepsy that reaches a peak around puberty and tends to disappear in adulthood.

The physician prescribed treatment. No further jerks or convulsions occurred and he did not have any side effects from the therapy.

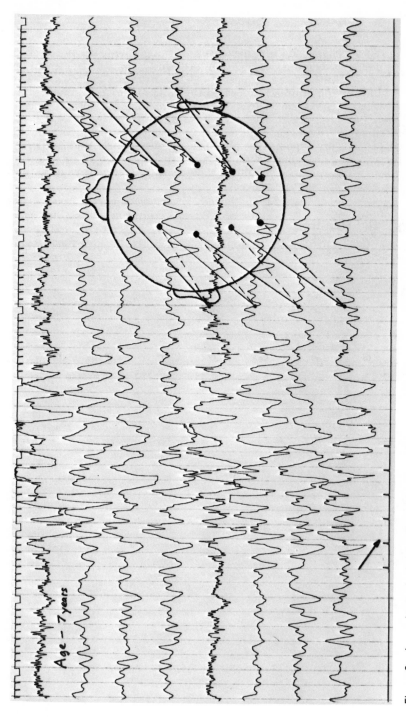

Figure 2. Intermittent photic stimulation of four flashes per second (see arrow) in this EEG precipitated an electrical discharge (photoconvulsive response). On this occasion the child with light-sensitive epilepsy did not have a seizure.

As a teenager, Ed's main concern was in getting a driver's license. He had to state on his application form that he was on treatment for epilepsy. The Registry requested a letter from his neurologist who again examined him and repeated the EEG. Although Ed never had any further convulsions or jerks, his EEG remained abnormal. During photic stimulation, however, when Ed was told to cover one eye, the tracing showed no abnormalities. The physician reassured him that he could drive, provided he took his medications regularly, and used some precautions, i.e., when driving against flickering lights, like on that Sunday afternoon, he should slow down and cover one eye until that dangerous stimulation is over.

Suggested Reading

Svoboda, W. B., 1979. Learning About Epilepsy. University Park Press, Baltimore.

chapter 5

Partial and Secondary Generalized Epilepsy

Partial (Focal) Epilepsy
Secondary Generalized Epilepsy
Differences and Similarities
Suggested Reading

Partial (Focal) Epilepsy

In partial (focal) epilepsy, the abnormal electrical discharges begin focally in one hemisphere and then may or may not spread to other areas of the brain. When consciousness is not affected, the epileptic attack is classified as simple partial seizure, and when it is impaired, complex partial seizure. That initial portion that occurs before consciousness is lost is called an *aura*. Sometimes auras are so short that the seizure seems to be generalized from the start. The usual causes are scarring due to different types of previous injury, certain forms of neurological disorders or rarely, a tumor. These causes are most often not inherited. Nevertheless, when an individual has a tendency to generalized seizures, after a head injury there is a higher chance of developing partial epilepsy.

The EEGs of children with partial epilepsy have one-sided "focal" electrical disturbances that are more readily visible in sleep. This is why so often sleep deprivation is necessary prior to the test in order for the child to fall asleep during the recording. Because the electrical abnormalities tend to spread quickly from their origin, the discharges may resemble those of generalized epilepsy. At other times the "focus" is far away from the surface of the brain. To discover "hidden sites," special electrodes (nasopharyngeal or sphenoidal) may need to be used to get closer to that abnormal area of cortex located in the base of the skull. Sometimes intravenous medications are given to "activate" the focal abnormality (see Chapter 3).

The importance of classifying epileptic attacks into two main groups (generalized and partial) is more than academic. Although a few anticonvulsant medications are good for both types of seizures, some are better than others. Furthermore, if exhaustive therapy fails to satisfactorily control partial seizures, brain surgery may be considered as alternative treatment in carefully selected individuals (see Chapter 8).

Benign Sylvian Seizures of Childhood

Rita Woods was a healthy 9-year-old—the youngest of three sisters. Early one morning she was suddenly awakened by the twitching of the right side of her face and her tongue felt like pins and needles. She sat up and saliva began to drool from the right corner of her mouth. Even though she was alert, Rita was unable to talk because she could not control her tongue. The attack lasted for a minute but her speech remained slurred for a short time. She had perfect recollection of the event and told her family. This strange episode did not make any sense to them and they did not take her to a physician. During the next 6 months three similar spells occurred. Then one morning the eldest sister was startled by the rhythmic knocking coming from Rita's bed and she saw that her body was shaking. Rita was having a convulsion.

She was admitted to hospital. All investigations were normal except the EEG. During drowsiness and sleep it showed a focal electrical discharge coming from the middle part of the left temporal lobe and the area slightly above it. The consulting neurologist diagnosed Sylvian seizure and prescribed treatment. He reassured the family that these children tend to respond well to medication and most often outgrow their attacks by the time they become teenagers. This is a form of epilepsy which is benign, usually appears between 8 and 10 years of age and disappears a few years later. The cause is hereditary but obscure.

Rita had no further seizures. At 15, when her EEG was normal, the treatment was stopped.

Complex Partial Seizures

Sixteen-year-old Sidney Johnson from Britain was visiting his relatives here when he had his first seizure. As he was chatting with his cousin, a sudden, strange, unexplainable, fearful feeling came over him. The next thing he remembered was that he was sitting on a bed, confused, tired, and somewhat nauseated, while his anxious relatives looked on. According to them he suddenly stopped talking and just stared ahead for a minute without moving; his eyes were lifeless, his face was pale, he kept swallowing and picking on his clothes. They shook him but he did not respond so, although he resisted, they led him to the nearest bed. After a minute, Sidney looked around, tried to say something but his words were slurred and did not make sense. He felt tired and drowsy but after a few minutes he was much better.

Sidney was upset. He tried to come up with an explanation so he said he probably had the flu. Two days later in the supermarket, an identical spell occurred. By this time his relatives realized that something very unusual was going on. They took Sidney to their family physician and he admitted him for investigations. Sidney's past history was normal in all respects. He was a healthy teenager, although he did have the occasional headache. The neurological examination was normal. His EEG, however, showed a left temporal lobe abnormality (focal slow wave disturbance) and because from his history there was no suggestion at all that Sidney should carry an old scar on his brain the doctors ordered further tests to rule out the possibility of an underlying tumor. A brain scan (CAT scan) identified a small mass in the left temporal lobe, which could well have represented a tumor. Exploratory surgery was recommended but his parents arranged for this to be done back in Britain.

Subsequent reports indicated that Sidney did have a slow growing benign tumor, which was fully removed. He had no further seizures.

The pattern of Sidney's epilepsy was typical of a kind of complex partial seizure originating from the temporal lobe.

Robert Donahue was 8 years old when he was hurt in school. He fell off a high wall and struck his head against a cement floor. Unconscious, he was taken by ambulance to the nearest hospital where x-rays showed a skull fracutre. Robert remained unconscious for 6 hours after which time he was irritable and lethargic for 5 or 6 days. Although the skull fracture healed, he was never the same. He could not concentrate well, was easily distracted by anything around him and the left side of his body was poorly coordinated; he developed a fine tremor in his hands. Robert needed special educational help to assist his learning and the family was heartbroken.

About a year after the accident, unexpectedly, Robert had a seizure. Following an unexplainable feeling he became confused and turned his head to the left while stretching out his right arm and right leg. He could vaguely hear his parents calling, "What is wrong?" but could not answer. The seizure lasted for a minute and it left him tired, confused, and fearful. Subsequently, an EEG showed an abnormality in the right frontal lobe—where the brunt of the injury occurred. Further tests revealed evidence of the widespread brain injury which led to the symptoms described.

Robert's life was greatly affected by his accident. He was always treated with a combination of two or three drugs but still his epilepsy was poorly controlled. He finished high school and became a machinist. One day during work he had a series of convulsions and lost his job. He retrained as an auto mechanic but due to his frequent seizures, he could not continue his employment.

Finally, after intensive investigations, it was decided to remove the most damaged part of the brain from where the seizures originated. The surgery was completed and although the seizures were much less frequent, Robert still had to take his anticonvulsant medications. How easily one's life can change through a sudden accident! Robert, also, had complex partial seizures originating from the frontal lobe.

In contrast to primary generalized convulsions in focal (partial) seizures, the abnormal electrical discharge begins in one region and then may or may not involve other areas and the entire brain. Depending on the origin and the spread, the symptoms and signs vary enormously. Sidney, for example, initially experienced a strange fearful feeling which was his warning (aura) and then he became confused, stared ahead, was pale, and kept swallowing (disturbance of autonomic behavior and of regulatory systems). Figure 1 shows the manifestations of focal seizures such as dizziness, nausea, hearing sounds, smelling unpleasant odors, visual illusions and hallucinations, feeling of numbness, twitching, and so on. Obviously, obtaining an accurate history in such epileptic attacks is crucial because it pinpoints the area of the brain that is involved in the disturbance. (See Chapter 9).

In contrast to Sidney's case, the vast majority of children do not have underlying tumors. In fact, most commonly the specific cause is not discovered even by detailed investigations. Occasionally it could be an injury to the brain in pregnancy, at birth, and perhaps later (as in Robert's case), or, it may be a focal developmental defect.

On rare occasions, older children seem to "talk" themselves out of their epileptic attacks by continuously saying something like this, "I am all right! I am all right!" Others can "walk their seizures off." If there is enough time after the warning they may go to the nearest chair, bed, or bathroom.

Walking aimlessly in a circle may at times be part of the epileptic attack. This type of epilepsy was originally named psychomotor seizure to indicate a combination of complex psychic sensations and stereotyped motor behavior. Such spells in most instances originate from the temporal lobe or its vicinity. The new International Classification System replaced this term with *complex partial seizures.* Anticonvulsant drugs alone or in combination frequently control these seizures.

Partial seizures (such as temporal lobe epilepsy) are difficult to tolerate. Often it is hard enough for adults and children to interpret their own normal reactions and feelings. For example, many students experience a strange discomfort or pain in their stomach before a test. It is a big step for them to recognize that the pain is a clue to the fact that they are worried and that they must study more. In other situations they may need to recognize a wish to be perfect, an underlying anger or other disguised or complicated thoughts and feelings. Now, this electrical disturbance may create new and troublesome sensations, memory and thought disturbance, speech arrest, fear, hallucinations, and illusions (Figure 1).

During the second decade of life, when temporal lobe epilepsy often begins, teenagers have more mature thinking abilities and more understanding of themselves and their families. This gives them a better chance to sort out additional problems and to manage some difficult periods. When the temporal lobe seizures are associated with episodes of irritability or impulses, most teenagers have learned how to channel and contain these feelings without causing increased disruption to themselves and others. Where this psychosocial learning has not been well formed, there is a higher risk of complications. (This learning is called psychosocial because it has two major components. The psychological component relates to how people learn about themselves, their emotions, and how to deal with them. The social component refers to acquiring interactional skills, how to assert oneself, how to share, compromise, and manage being angry and so on. Most of these negotiating abilities are first learned in the family.) Usually when a child and family have had difficulty learning to communicate and deal with feelings, psychosocial help is required along with appropriate medical care.

Partial seizures may pose particular difficulties for younger children because they lack the diverse experience of the teenager and are less aware of how to manage difficult feelings. Because the symptoms can include cognitive problems (disturbance of thinking) and displays of unusual behavior or emotions, the family is faced with additional stress. The parents must understand "what is what" at first before they can sympathetically begin to help their children increase their coping skills.

A further complication for youngsters who have focal seizures is that the onset of epilepsy may be associated with some degree of hyperactivity. This means that their ability to attend is decreased, they may be irritable, impulsive, restless, and energetic without seeming to be able to direct their activity appropriately. Their learning may also be affected. These additional symptoms pose an extra task for parents. Behavioral guidelines, the structure in the home, and increased communication all need to be augmented in order to continue to foster the positive development of these children. An excellent parenting book has been written by Stewart and Olds (1973) on the management of hyperactivity.

When a seizure disorder is associated with altered behavior, parents are often particularly confused because they relate it to changes in the child's EEG. How can they discipline an electrical discharge? Parents, like their children with epilepsy, can find it difficult to distinguish between "seizure behavior" and misbehavior. Seizures can leave a person tired, inattentive, confused, agitated, and unpredictable for several hours or even longer. In such situations, the ability to perceive what is happening and what is bad behavior may be clouded but not lost. The children's fragile state of control, however, needs all the support it can get. Parents should set "limits with love" and use just one set of rules for behavior disturbance due to seizures and for being naughty; otherwise, these children become confused. Their "seizure misbehavior" can become worse without clear limits. Even when parents are absolutely certain that the irritability from seizures increases their misbehavior, limits still are needed. Children need to learn to behave appropriately even when they don't feel well. Rules can be modulated, not changed. For example, when a seizure makes them irritable and naughty the rule is still the loss of television privileges but not for the whole evening. It is possible to tell them that "because you feel bad, it is harder to keep your temper. You still need to remember the rules. Because you were yelling you will miss one program on television tonight." Allowing them to take it out on the home or on the family does not prepare them for getting along with others in the future (see Chapter 13).

Somatosensory Partial Seizures ("Jacksonian March")

John Powers is a 17-year-old high school student who is regularly seen at the seizure clinic. In his early childhood he was involved in a car accident. A truck hit the side of the family car and John sustained a concussion. He was unconscious for about 30 minutes but there were no other apparent complications. About a year later, he developed focal seizures which sometimes led to generalized convulsions. Doctors tried several anticonvulsants; Tegretol proved to be the most satisfactory although occasionally mild seizures occurred.

The attacks always began in the left hand. First an odd indescribable, warm sensation appeared in his fingers followed in 5–10 seconds by the feeling of pins and needles. The sensation then spread up his arm and simultaneously to the left side of his face. Occasionally, he also experienced some twitching in his left arm and face but if the seizure went beyond this point he lost consciousness and had a generalized convulsion. However, since the treatment with Tegretol was started the seizure never progressed into a generalized convulsion.

John quite accidentally found a way to prevent the abnormal feeling from traveling. He noticed that when the odd warmness first appeared in his fingers, if he squeezed them hard enough or repeatedly shook them, the seizure disappeared. With this method and the Tegretol therapy his seizure control was quite satisfactory.

John's attacks represent a rare form of focal seizure disorder. As the electrical discharges over the sensorimotor cortex of the right hemisphere slowly spread, his symptoms also changed. This type of epilepsy is called *Jacksonian March*. Some individuals, by their own specific technique, can prevent its progression. It is not understood why this is possible in some kinds of seizures and not in others. John's initial attacks are classified as simple partial seizures because his consciousness is not impaired, but before anticonvulsant treatment they sometimes progressed to secondarily generalized convulsions.

Special Sensory (Occipital Lobe) Seizures

Paul Murphy, a 10-year-old, was born after a long difficult labor which ended up in an emergency Caesarean section. His motor coordination was always poor. When he was in grade one a learning disability became apparent.

Several times during the past year Paul complained to his mother about seeing colored spots. These appeared to be whirling several feet before his left eye and for perhaps half a minute. They disappeared as abruptly as they came, leaving Paul with a vague headache for 1 to 2 hours. The parents first felt that this was eyestrain but the ophthalmologist did not find anything wrong. Several months passed by and Paul continued having these spells, usually late in the afternoon and quite often before bedtime. Then on one occasion the episode lasted longer. Paul became confused, stared ahead with a vacant look and his left arm jerked a few times. He was very tired afterwards and just wanted to sleep. Next day the worried parents went to their family physician who made the tentative diagnosis of a seizure disorder and referred Paul to a child neurologist.

The neurological examination showed only some minor coordination problems but the EEG was abnormal. During drowsiness and more so in sleep, a frequently discharging spike focus appeared over the right occipital lobe. Now everything fitted the diagnosis. Paul had occipital lobe seizures. When he was tired and sleepy often just prior to his bedtime, the electrical abnormality became active causing the occasional sudden visual hallucinations. During the last episode, however, the discharge must have spread to other areas of the brain, making Paul confused. Although the epilepsy emerged late, the cause was felt to be the difficult birth. The CAT scan showed slight enlargement of the ventricles which was interpreted as evidence of minimal but diffuse damage to the hemispheres.

Even though the seizures were minor they responded poorly to anticonvulsant therapy. After several drug trials the spells subsided on Tegretol and Dilantin.

Secondary Generalized Epilepsy

In contrast to idiopathic *primary* generalized epilepsy the type of generalized seizures discussed here are *secondary*. They are caused or accompanied frequently by severe and diffuse disorders of the brain (encephalopathy). Such encephalopathies may be produced by a hidden smoldering viral infection that is not apparent on tests like a spinal tap. It has been speculated that as sometimes kidneys or the thyroid gland become the target of a self-directed autoimmune disease, the brain could be damaged in a similar process. Nevertheless, the cause is obscure in most instances.

The epileptic attacks in this group are usually generalized but sometimes they show characteristic features of frontal and temporal lobe seizures. Children, during their absence spells, may look dazed but are still responsive to calls in contrast to petit mal. Therefore, these seizures are called *incomplete* or *atypical absence spells.* When having convulsions, only the stiffening (the tonic phase) may be present whereas the twitching (the clonic phase) is minimal or not apparent at all.

In a classic grand mal convulsion, as discussed in Chapter 4, the stiffening phase is always followed by twitching. The secondarily generalized seizures tend to be shorter than in idiopathic forms of epilepsy. Often they are limited to a brief, simple body jerk, which is called a *myoclonic seizure,* or to a few seconds of body stiffening, classified as a *tonic seizure.* Still these children lose their balance and hurt themselves. Similar drop attacks could also be caused by a sudden loss of muscle tone or strength in which case the spells are described as *atonic seizures.* In atonic seizures the fall is more gradual than in myoclonic and tonic seizures but serious injuries may occur. Drop attacks are also known as *astatic seizures* (loss of stance) or as *akinetic seizures* (loss of motion) because after falling, some of the children may remain motionless and floppy for a variable period of time. Obviously, the large number of terms that describe the various forms of epilepsy can cause confusion. The exact classification, however, is not only useful to physicians but also to parents who need to understand the underlying mechanisms leading to these attacks and to realize the complexity of the neurological disorder affecting their children.

During these seizures the change of consciousness is hardly apparent because their duration is so brief, the post-ictal effects are minimal and recovery is immediate. Nevertheless, the attacks may be frequent and so unexpected that wearing a protective helmet is often warranted.

Individuals with myoclonic or atonic spells in the daytime may have frequent tonic seizures in their sleep. *Nocturnal* (night) *seizures* are just as brief as those in wakefulness and can be easily confused with ordinary stretching. They are not dangerous but when very frequent, the pattern of sleep is disturbed and the children are exhausted the next day.

Children with "incomplete absences" may seem dazed and yet their seizures may be overlooked until there is a slight head drop or a tendency to fall forward. Their EEGs show diffuse abnormalities similar to those of petit mal but more irregular. In addition, the electrical discharges (slow spike-waves) are virtually continuous, therefore, the brain is in a state of constant turmoil. Response to the environment is greatly reduced, although almost never totally lost, the motions are slow and the ability to process new information is impaired. Considerable psychomotor retardation is commonly present. Placement in special classes for slow learners is often necessary. Academic progress is slow and the developmental gap tends to increase every year.

The mechanisms of the various seizures and the intellectual impairment are poorly understood. It is not clear whether the arrest or lack of progress is related to the seizures or if both are the result of a nonspecified encephalopathy.

Treatment is not always satisfactory. At times, an anticonvulsant improves one type of seizure but makes the other worse. Most often several drugs are necessary, leading to the danger of more side effects. Major convulsions are often prevented but the therapy has little influence on the minor ones. Exacerbations alternate with remissions, which seem to become longer with age. It is estimated that at least two-thirds of these children will eventually stop having seizures. A variable degree of intellectual deficit, however, remains in most instances.

A well-balanced combination of anticonvulsants and multidisciplinary support helps overcome difficult times. The concentrated efforts of the family, teachers, counselors, and others are necessary to prevent such children from becoming socially isolated by the time they reach adolescence when the seizures are often less severe or no longer represent a problem.

Infantile Spasms

Mrs. Kovacs brought her 5-month-old son to the clinic at the suggestion of the family physician. Steven had been a healthy infant until the last 2 to 3 weeks when he was having frequent sudden body jerks and also seemed less responsive than before. During the examination he abruptly swung his arms across his chest, pulled his knees up over his stomach, then relaxed a second later. The pattern was so typical that the diagnosis was immediately apparent—Steven had infantile spasms. A subsequent EEG confirmed this impression. A CAT scan showed multiple calcified areas in the brain, which was diagnostic of tuberous sclerosis. This explained the cause of seizures.

Steven's parents took the diagnosis hard when they were told the high chance for mental retardation. They were given articles to read in addition to the repeated discussions carried on with them. Treatment did not completely stop the spasms but seizures disappeared by the age of 3. Still, at 5, Steven's development was only at the level of 18 months. As time went on, he was seen by a psychologist who evaluated his learning capabilities. A speech therapist recommended language stimulation and he was enrolled in a special preschool. In case they decided to have more children, the parents were counseled about the chances of tuberous sclerosis occurring again. This chance was small in their case and they now have a healthy 2-year-old girl. The Kovacs family experienced hard times but, with supportive help, they managed.

Recently, April Hallum, a 6-month-old infant who had just developed infantile spasms, was referred to the seizure clinic. Her development until that time was satisfactory. Although the neurological examination was normal, the EEG showed a hypsarrhythmic pattern. Therapy with steroids (ACTH and subsequently prednisone) began immediately and within a few days the seizures disappeared. The EEG also became normal. A CAT scan was done and it revealed no abnormalities. After 6 months the medication was gradually discontinued. The infantile spasms did not return and repeated EEG's remained normal. Developmentally, April is still doing well. It was felt that the early diagnosis and immediate therapy contributed to the successful outcome.

Infantile spasms occur almost exclusively in infancy. The disorder is also known by a variety of descriptive terms, such as, massive myoclonic jerks, salaam seizures, jack-knife convulsions, among others. They are characterized by a sudden stiffening of the body and the infant momentarily loses contact with the environment. Depending on which part of the body is involved in the spasm, head nodding, doubling up, sudden stretching of the arms and legs or simply eye rolling may be seen. Initially only occasional spasms occur throughout the day and they are not infrequently mistaken for colic because during the spells, gas may be expelled. Later the seizures come in groups ("showers") mainly after awakening from sleep or a nap. Many of these infants show evidence of previous brain damage or a neurological disorder (like Steven) while others seem to have been entirely normal until the onset of seizures (like April). The EEG is usually markedly abnormal, often showing the so-called characteristic hypsarrhythmic pattern (Figure 1).

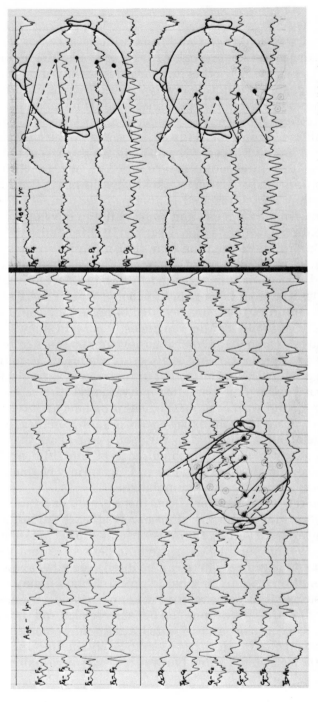

Figure 1. A hypsarrhythmic EEG on the left. The infant has infantile spasms. The EEG on the right is that of a normal child in the same age group.

The treatment is difficult and some infants may not respond well to such drugs as intramuscular ACTH, steroids, Mogadon, Clonopin, and Depakene. The other anticonvulsants have no influence on infantile spasms. It is not clear why the medications are effective in some infants but not in others. Those with no pre-existing brain damage as in April's case have a greater chance of success. The majority of children become mentally retarded even when the seizures are controlled and this fact is very difficult for the parents to face. The cause of this intellectual deterioration is obscure. Infantile spasms spontaneously disappear, usually by the age of 2 or 3 years even when they fail to respond to therapy. Unfortunately, other types of seizures may appear and some children develop Lennox-Gastaut syndrome, which is also described in this chapter.

It is appropriate to mention here that infantile spasms are a common early manifestation of tuberous sclerosis. This inherited neurological disease is characterized by the presence of multiple small nodules scattered throughout the body. When a CAT scan of the brain is obtained, these are revealed because they contain calcium, usually adjacent to the ventricles. The skin shows white patches, and later an unusual rash also develops on the face. Mental retardation and various types of seizures are common. The manifestations and prognosis of this disorder are extremely variable; therefore, each case needs to be evaluated individually.

Having a child with a major medical problem can have a profound impact. Apart from the experience of assault, complex feelings often emerge about family origins, the spouse and about the future. Reality questions about the medical care of the child are compounded by confusion, guilt, and anger. Uncertainty begins to be a daily experience, and it can be immobilizing.

This type of problem never affects just the mother or the father. Both sets of grandparents are often involved, each giving advice from totally different vantage points. A friendship network—if it includes other young parents—can vacillate between attentive support and fearful distance. There can be intense debates about how much information to share or what to reveal. Isolation may be preferred to disappointing some relative with an irritable response on a bad day. None of these questions can be easily settled and they often require much discussion and repeated attention. Something that seems settled on one day does not seem to be on another. In spite of the fact that discussion is often painful, it proves invaluable in the long run.

Lennox-Gastaut Syndrome

Four-year-old Peter was the only child of Mr. and Mrs. Welsh who married late. The mother was a school teacher and the father a contractor. Their main enjoyment in life was Peter, a bright, charming little boy.

Early in March, unexpectedly, Peter had a short generalized convulsion for which he was admitted to a hospital and a diagnosis of epilepsy was made. In spite of phenobarbital therapy, he had more seizures. These were different; at breakfast, his head would suddenly fall forward two or three times. These episodes did not tire him out as had the first grand mal convulsion—in fact, Mrs. Welsh was not certain if they were seizures. She took him to the family physician, who suggested further observation. The head drops occurred more and more frequently and then Peter began falling forward, sometimes hitting his head against the floor. He had to wear a hockey helmet for protection. His concentration span was now shorter and he became fidgety. Mrs. Welsh, with the keen eye of a school teacher, sensed that Peter's intellectual progress had slowed down.

After more investigations, the heartbroken parents observed yet another type of seizure during which Peter stared ahead for 10 to 20 seconds and then was tired. Often the staring was accompanied by slight head bobbing or head falling. Nothing could get him out of these spells although at times after calling or shaking he seemed to respond somewhat by turning around with a vacant look. In September, the diagnosis of Lennox-Gastaut syndrome was made. It was difficult to fully explain to the parents what this disorder was as even physicians do not fully understand it. Peter was treated with Depakene and Tegretol. His seizure control was good although occasionally seizures did occur.

The syndrome was named after two epileptologists, Lennox and Gastaut. It is grouped into two types. In one there is pre-existing, often severe, diffuse brain damage usually dating back to pregnancy or birth. Many of these children have infantile spasms in infancy from which they recover but after a seizure-free period they start all over again with a more complex seizure pattern.

In the other form, as in Peter's case, the development is normal during the first few years of life. The onset for both groups is usually between the ages of 2 and 5 years. The cause is severe brain damage in the first type but in the second it is obscure. Children who are normal prior to the onset of seizures frequently slow down intellectually. Perhaps this deterioration is caused by a not apparent infection of the brain that may be a virus.

Characteristically, there is a wide variety of seizures that do not fall into the stereotyped categories described above. These children may just be staring vacantly or stiffen out briefly with rapid blinking. They may have myoclonic seizures (a sudden jerk, a head drop, a sudden fall) or other types with even less defined patterns. Major convulsions occur less frequently, usually are shorter than typical grand mal attacks, and are not followed by post-ictal depression. The above described patterns are in many ways very troublesome because they can be extremely frequent and may interfere with the child's behavior and performance. The seizures can virtually go on day and night—usually fleeting absence spells and drop attacks during wakefulness while tonic or tonic-clonic seizures in sleep. No wonder these children will be functioning poorly during these times.

Fortunately, exacerbation of seizure activity is followed by periods of relative quiescence. Commonly a fall in anticonvulsant blood levels explains the deterioration, although not infrequently the reason remains obscure. On the other hand, decreasing or even eliminating some of the medications, especially the least effective ones, often helps to reduce the number of epileptic attacks. Probably this is because such change alleviates some of the side effects. Among those, drowsiness in particular should be avoided because it tends to facilitate seizures. Children who are active and alert (in contrast to being inactive) have less frequent seizures. The reason for this may be difficult for parents to understand. Earlier in the book, the function of the brain was compared to an orchestra. At the beginning the musicians start out by practicing different notes so the music sounds chaotic. As soon as the conductor activates the orchestra by tapping his baton, all musicians begin to work together. There is no longer any disorganization. Similarly, when children with Lennox-Gastaut syndrome or other types of epilepsy are alerted, their EEGs often show an immediate reduction in the frequency and extent of abnormal electrical discharges. Healthy activity as compared to idleness reduces the chance of seizures.

The EEG, which is always abnormal, shows very frequent slow spike and wave discharges, usually spreading to all regions of the brain (Figure 2). Contrary to petit mal, the discharges are present even when these children do not show any evidence of seizures. They are slow but responsive and do not have any twitching. The electrical abnormalities are greatly increased in sleep, but curiously, they almost disappear during active dreaming. The EEG is abnormal between the discharges and tends to remain so even when the seizures eventually become controlled, for example, in adolescence. Likewise, behavior and cognitive functions will always be impaired. A multidisciplinary approach with neurologists, psychologists, nurses, social workers, and teachers joining forces in the care of these children is most helpful for the parents.

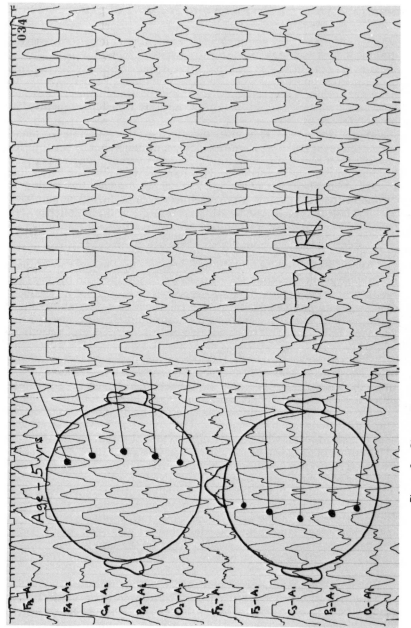

Figure 2.   Slow spike and wave discharges in Lennox-Gastaut Syndrome.

Myoclonic—Absence Seizures and Hyperactivity

David Bennett was the youngest of three healthy children. At birth the umbilical cord was found to be tightly twisted around his neck. During the first year of life he was irritable but still played quietly with his toys, sometimes for hours. However, from the moment he learned to walk, his behavior became hyperactive. All day he raced around, jumping up and down on furniture and even though he hurt himself frequently, he hardly ever cried.

When David was 20 months old, during a flu epidemic, he developed high fever and had a 3-minute long convulsion but by the time his parents took him to the hospital he had recovered. Blood tests and a lumbar puncture were normal and the parents were told that David had the flu. A couple of days later his EEG showed generalized bursts of "irregular spike and slow wave discharges" both during wakefulness and sleep—the type of abnormality seen in generalized epilepsy. The family physician prescribed phenobarbital but it was discontinued because it made David's hyperactive behavior worse. Another anticonvulsant was not given and he had no further convulsion.

At 3, David could say only a few words and expressed himself mainly by gestures although he appeared to comprehend his parents. At around this time his EEG was repeated. It showed more frequent discharges now and some of them were associated with eyeblinking or slight body jerks which were not very noticeable. He continued to have frequent falls, thought to be related to his hurried and impulsive behavior.

When he was 4 years old, David was enrolled in a special nursery school to provide him with a structured environment. His teacher noticed that several times a day he stopped for a couple of seconds, blinked, rolled his eyes back and then he would return to his previous chaotic overactivity. During these episodes he did not seem to understand directions and his responses, if any, were inappropriate. He was sent to a neurologist who began anticonvulsant treatment, but in spite of a number of drug combinations his seizures continued. At this stage he was referred to a specialized seizure clinic. There, David's EEG and behavior were simultaneously analyzed through video-tape recordings while he was allowed to play. The frequent electrical discharges were associated with minimal absence seizures as described by the teacher. During his brief "staring spells" sometimes his arms were shaken by a few subtle jerks. After these episodes when he was quiet, his hyperactive behavior returned with a sudden burst. His actions were irrational, he was ready to bite and just wandered around aimlessly until the next seizure.

As a first step in the treatment, much of the unnecessary medication was discontinued. Eventually his seizures were better controlled by a now rarely used old drug called Tridione and he became more responsive. His behavior improved further by using a stimulant drug, Ritalin; nevertheless he needed to continue his education in a special class.

Hyperactive children, like David, do best in a controlled, structured environment. They cannot tolerate any excess stimulation because their attention span is so short and they are too easily distracted. David's behavior was further disrupted by his recurring seizures. This case report is representative of a group of children who are born with some kind of brain damage resulting in marked behavioral difficulties. When seizures appear, some of them will develop Lennox-Gastaut Syndrome and become retarded in their further development. Others, like David, will have only a very subtle type of epilepsy, myoclonic-absence seizures, which makes them more disruptive and often uncontrollably aggressive.

Differences and Similarities

It is surprising that a medical condition such as epilepsy can take on so many different forms. It may even seem contradictory that absence seizures (petit mal) and primary generalized convulsions (grand mal) belong to the same group and that the opposite manifestations of stiffening and falling limp (tonic and atonic seizures) can occur in the same individual at different times of the day. Also surprising is why a similar grand mal attack can be the expression of a seizure disorder with or without encephalopathy. The answer to these questions comes from an understanding of how the brain is built and organized (see Chapter 3). Nerve cells generate electrical signals (discharges) that in normal conditions carry useful messages. Electricity travels along conductors even at great distance (the power lines), likewise it moves along predisposed pathways outside and within the brain.

The circuitries in the nervous system are designed with great precision to execute a multitude of functions and to transmit information from one point to another. All this is accomplished, like in modern electronic microdevices, with incredible economy of space and simplicity. For instance, the electrical signal carrying a pleasurable or painful sensation from one organ to the brain is always the same in quality and intensity. Nevertheless, the sensation is perceived differently according to the number of signals fired, to the location of the terminals in the organ and depending where in the brain such signals are received. In addition, because the pathways in the nervous system are so closely packed, if for some abnormal reason the number of signals fired at the same time exceed certain limits, a chain reaction may be triggered. Now the sparkles that were supposed to keep the engine running with great precision become an explosion shuttering the whole system. That is how seizures begin, and once started, this avalanche of energy is shunted so that not only regular pathways but also unusual connections are excited.

This mechanism explains why an electrical seizure in the occipital lobe may cause perception of visual images that are not there. This may be followed by a multitude of other hallucinatory experiences if the memory storage in the temporal lobe becomes involved. A variety of posturing and movement may occur if the electrical discharge spreads to parts of the cortex in the frontal lobe, which control motor activity. Such progression and continuity of functions is rationally predetermined and is an essential part of normal brain organization. When the spread of signals becomes tumultuous and uncontrolled, however, the functions become unbalanced, and the behavior irrational. Such breakdowns can be called *seizures* because now the system is controlled by these abnormal forces that normally should serve the system.

Understandably, seizures can vary greatly because there are so many functions represented in the brain. At the same time, because the different areas of the central nervous system are so intimately interconnected, one type of seizure can evolve into another.

If one part of the brain is abnormal, the seizures will always start there and due to the consistent origin and pattern of spread, the manifestations will remain rather stereotyped for that individual. It is important to note that there are not only excitatory but also inhibitory signals that control functions by dampening excitation. The inhibitor systems are as widespread as the excitatory ones and they are equally essential. They represent a natural defense against seizures because their presence may be a barrier to the spread of abnormal discharges. For instance, experiencing an "aura" without going into a full convulsion means exactly that. There are medications that are effective by decreasing excitation and others by increasing inhibition (see Chapter 7). An inborn deficiency of the inhibitory system is believed to be one of the main reasons why individuals with idiopathic epilepsy have a greater predisposition to seizures.

Finally all areas of the cortex must be connected by direct pathways to the centers in order to promote self-awareness; otherwise, all cognitive functions would not be conscious experiences. The system of awareness is a diffuse network of nerve cells in the deep core of the brain. It is in constant interplay with each hemisphere above and with centers of the spinal cord below. This explains why an unrestrained explosion of electrical discharges starting either in the deep core of the brain (generalized epilepsies) or spreading to it from any other area of the cortex (partial epilepsy with secondary generalization) will have the same consequences. They abolish consciousness and cause massive motor activity through bombarding the centers of muscle control in the spinal cord (grand mal). The difference between a grand mal and a petit mal is the involvement or non-involvement of these spinal cord centers. In both there is loss of consciousness, the site of origin is the core of the brain but the pattern of spread differs with remarkable consequences.

Within the spinal cord, like in the higher parts of the brain there are two systems. One sends excitatory and the other inhibitory signals. They are separate although working in synchrony and are closely connected. In special circumstances, the electrical discharges that are carried from the brain to the periphery, may be channeled through either one with the opposite results. A massive muscle contraction (tonic seizure) or a loss of muscle tone (atonic seizure) may occur.

Epilepsy is quite a kaleidoscopic condition that reflects the marvelous organization of the brain. The seizures represent a breakdown or an exaggeration of normal functions. Epilepsy is, therefore, not a single disorder but the expression of a great variety of diseases and conditions with or without a lesion in the brain. Knowledge of the epileptic manifestations is of great interest because it discloses the nature and the location of the underlying disorder.

Suggested Reading

Stewart, M. A., and Olds, S. W. 1973. Raising a Hyperactive Child. Harper & Row, New York.

chapter 6

What Is Not Epilepsy?

Febrile Seizures
Hypnogogic Jerks, Twitches during Sleep, and Startling
Night Terrors
Migraine Headaches
Temper Tantrums
Daydreaming
Tics and Jerks
Fainting
Pallid Syncope
Breath-holding Spells
Psychogenic Epilepsy

If a child has seizures, usually the parents quickly learn the pattern of the attacks. Not infrequently a number of complaints may be associated and confused with epilepsy. Unexplained falls, temper tantrums, breath-holding spells, migraine headaches, dizziness, fainting, night terrors, daydreaming, restless sleep, and tics may be noticed and worry the parents. These common disorders are described in this chapter so that parents can understand them better and learn what makes them different from epilepsy. Febrile seizures are also discussed here because most of them are not considered to be true epilepsy.

Febrile Seizures

Eighteen-month-old Dedra McQuinn developed a cold with a burning fever. Two hours later during her nap, she suddenly startled and then her body began to jerk rhythmically for about a minute. The parents immediately called their family physician who arrived 20 minutes later. By that time Dedra was resting peacefully. Although this was Dedra's first convulsion, Mrs. McQuinn was not alarmed since her older daughter and her nephew both had had one or two similar seizures during febrile illnesses in their early childhood.

The family physician, after making a careful physical examination and taking into consideration the strong family history of febrile seizures concluded that Dedra had a febrile seizure but he did not feel that immediate hospitalization was necessary. He discussed the indications for anticonvulsant therapy but postponed it until she could be fully evaluated at the seizure clinic. He gave treatment for the cold and instructed the parents on how to keep down the temperature. Since he did not completely rule out meningitis the doctor phoned back several times and asked to see Dedra in his office the next day—just to make sure there were no problems.

At the seizure clinic all investigations, including an EEG, were normal and the diagnosis of a simple febrile convulsion was made. After careful consideration it was decided not to start Dedra's phenobarbital therapy.

The McQuinn family was fortunate in having such a conscientious physician; nowadays few make house calls in large cities, preferring rather to meet their patients at the hospital emergency where additional equipment is available if needed.

Late at night, after 2-year-old Jennifer Toner's birthday party, she developed a severe earache with a temperature of 105° F. As she lay crying on her mother's lap she became strangely quiet for several seconds. Suddenly her right arm and leg rhythmically began to jerk, gradually spreading to the other side. By now Jennifer was unconscious, very pale, and her eyes were rolled back. Mrs. Toner noticed that the twitching was more marked on the right side of the body. The father called the ambulance and when it arrived 10 minutes later the convulsion was still going strong. As the ambulance sped toward the hospital the twitching subsided, first on the left side and after a few strong jerks it disappeared also on the right. Jennifer was in a deep sleep. All this was very frightening for the parents, especially since no one in the family, including Jennifer, had ever before had a seizure.

The nurses in the emergency room notified the family physician who immediately asked a pediatrician for a consultation. After a careful physical examination the ear infection was diagnosed. Since the cause of this approximately 25-minute long convulsion was still unclear, meningitis (bacterial infection of the brain) had to be ruled out. The doctor explained that just the other day he had treated a child with a temperature and seizures who turned out to have meningitis and needed immediate intravenous antibiotic therapy.

Fortunately, in Jennifer's case the analysis of the spinal fluid was normal. She was kept in hospital and her treatment with antibiotics for the ear infection started. Next day the EEG showed only nonspecific findings and she was feeling better. The physicians who were looking after Jennifer concluded that she had had an atypical complex febrile seizure and they decided to prescribe phenobarbital therapy for about 2 years. The parents were instructed in how to keep the temperature down during febrile illnesses and they were given an office appointment for a follow-up visit.

Febrile seizures are most commonly seen between the ages of 6 months and 3 years. They are generally brief, usually of less than 15 minutes, and tend to occur during the first day of illness, particularly during the period of rapid temperature rise. Most commonly the temperature of the child at the time of convulsion or immediately after is above 101° F. Frequently other members of the family also had convulsions with high fever in their early childhood. These are known as simple febrile convulsions.

A febrile seizure is defined as atypical or complex when it occurs frequently; the associated temperature is lower than 101°–102° F.; the convulsive part lasts longer than 15 minutes and only one side of the body is involved or remains weak after the episode is over; the EEG, the neurological examination, or development are not normal;

and when there is no family history of similar spells. However, it is not always easy to separate simple febrile convulsions from complex ones. There are exceptions. For example, occasionally a simple febrile convulsion can be quite long, and in very young children the seizure may involve only one side of the body. The cause is not entirely clear. Children with simple febrile seizures seem to have inherited a predisposition to convulsions that are precipitated by high fever only during early childhood. This may be frightening but simple febrile convulsions are not life threatening and are almost universally considered to be a benign condition. Many physicians feel that prophylactic treatment is not required.

In contrast, the brain of children with complex febrile seizures may contain other underlying precipitating mechanisms that predispose to convulsions; therefore, anticonvulsant treatment with phenobarbital and more recently with Depakene is frequently recommended. The EEG does not necessarily have to be abnormal before considering therapy if one or more of the atypical features outlined above are present. These triggers may become apparent only as the child grows beyond the age of 4–6 years when the tendency for simple febrile convulsion has diminished. The risk of developing one form of epilepsy or another seems to be statistically much greater with complex than with simple febrile seizures.

To protect children from recurrent febrile seizures, parents and doctors are frequently faced with the dilemma of starting them on medications that could cause side effects or just trying to prevent the temperature from rising very high. This may be difficult to do during the night when everyone is asleep but these pros and cons should be openly and carefully discussed. The parents need to be comfortable with the plan. Once treatment is initiated, it may be continued until the children seem to have outgrown their predisposition, but this decision is obviously influenced by a number of variables.

Although there is and probably always will be some controversy about the need for prophylactic treatment, the elevated temperature of a child with the diagnosis of febrile seizures must be quickly reduced. First, the body is exposed, then it is covered with a wet (not ice cold) cloth so that the evaporating water can bring down the fever. In addition, fanning can speed up this cooling process. Ice cold baths or showers and ice water enemas should not be used. After "sponging," appropriate doses of aspirin or Tylenol are given to keep the temperature down for longer periods of time. Too much of these drugs is harmful; therefore, parents should carefully follow the directions. It is also very useful to give frequent sips of favorite ice-cold drinks. Even icicles will help bring down the temperature. As has already been emphasized, phenobarbital given after the fever develops is ineffective because it takes several days for it to reach sufficiently high concentration in the brain to prevent the occurrence of febrile seizures.

Hypnogogic Jerks, Twitches during Sleep, and Startling

Most people have experienced a sudden momentary twitch of the body just before falling asleep. Also, particularly during dreams, little random muscle twitches of the face, arms, and legs normally occur. In addition, when an infant is awakened or surprised by a loud noise, he or she reacts with a characteristic startle response, a sudden outflinging of the arms. All these involuntary muscle jerks are normal but sometimes parents of children with epilepsy mistake them for seizure activity. In case of uncertainty, a sleep EEG will resolve the issue.

Night Terrors

Night terrors, which are mainly a disorder of children, occur suddenly in the middle of the night. The children scream and thrash around in great disarray and confusion. They may seem awake but do not recognize their parents and are hard to console. Gradually, in a few minutes or longer, the youngsters stop crying, relax, and fall back to sleep. The next morning they cannot recall the events. These are frightening episodes for the parents but not for the child. They can occur more than once during the same night and several times a week. Recently it has been shown that night terror is not a bad dream or an epileptic disorder but rather a specific sleep disturbance, a sudden incomplete arousal from sleep. If "medical" treatment is desired, medication given at bedtime may abolish this disorder. Eventually, with or without medicine, it spontaneously subsides. Children should stay in their own rooms. Adjustments or the addition of anticonvulsant drugs are not necessary. Occasionally even experienced child neurologists have difficulty differentiating night terrors from seizures and are forced to request an all-night electroencephalogram with monitoring of respiration, heart rate, eye movement, and muscle tone. This helps to clarify the diagnosis.

Migraine Headaches

Migraine headache is usually a benign condition and is easily diagnosed. Atypical forms though can be confused with epilepsy. In the absence of a specific diagnostic test for migraine, the final proof is based primarily on the history.

The "classical" migraine headache is characterized by severe, throbbing pain above one or both eyes, associated with nausea and vomiting. Before the onset the child may experience a period of visual, auditory, or sensory disturbances (prodrome). Often zig-zag colored silvery lines or a black spot, or both, appear in one half of the visual fields. Things may seem to be getting smaller or bigger, sounds can be louder or muffled, and numbness or pinpricks in one part of the body may also appear. Rarely, one side of the body is temporarily weak or numb (hemiplegic migraine).

It is believed that these symptoms are caused by constriction of some of the arteries in the brain, which reduces the flow of blood; subsequently the arteries dilate and that produces the headache. Noise, strong light, or movement exacerbate the pain. When the individual vomits, the headache improves and may soon subside. Usually, there is a strongly positive history of similar disturbances in other family members. Not infrequently in children the headache represents a minimal component and the whole attack may consist of the preceding symptoms especially stomach complaints. Such episodes may resemble some types of temporal lobe epilepsy. Like seizures, these atypical migraine symptoms may come and go quickly. Contrary to epilepsy, consciousness is not impaired during an attack of migraine. These individuals can describe lucidly and in great detail their experiences and can become very apprehensive about them.

There is a form of migraine during which the child becomes confused, weak, or dizzy. On extremely rare occasions the person may even fall to the ground unconscious and could have a brief convulsion. Such children are often referred to neurologists and a diagnosis is reached only after extensive investigations.

The nature of migraine, even more so than epilepsy, is poorly understood. Both present many analogies and not infrequently overlap. Consequently it is difficult to draw the line between the two disorders. To make it more confusing, some of the medications that effectively prevent migraine in children are the same as used for epilepsy. As a rule, one should remember that epileptic attacks are caused by excessive electrical discharge originating from the "abnormal" parts of the brain whereas migraine seems to represent the response of normal brain to spasms of arteries. Not all recurrent headaches are migraine. Sometimes, especially when they wake a child up, it is advisable for the parents to obtain a neurological consultation.

Temper Tantrums

Children with epilepsy can have temper tantrums just like other youngsters. On the other hand, tantrums may be mistakenly viewed as a form of seizures, especially temporal lobe epilepsy.

> Chris was born 9 weeks prematurely and had some difficulties as a newborn. His motor and language development were impaired but his intelligence was normal. At the age of 5 he experienced two generalized convulsions for which he was treated with Dilantin; he had no further seizures.
>
> When Chris was 8 years old, with increasing frequency, he began to have "unprovoked" rage attacks. During these episodes he smashed everything he could put his hands on, kicked, scratched, and bit anyone close by. His eyes were glazed, his face red and perspiring. The attacks occurred at home and to the embarrassment of the parents, in crowded department stores, on the playground, in school, and even in church. After several minutes of forceful restriction he relaxed and then curled up for a short nap. After one such episode, his mother took him to the family physician who suggested that this might be temporal lobe epilepsy and added phenobarbital. This made him even more restless (a common side effect of phenobarbital) and his rages persisted. By this time Chris had been transferred into a Special Class because the risk of another child getting hurt was too great. The school requested detailed neurological and psychiatric evaluations.
>
> The psychological tests and psychiatric interviews showed that because of his significant learning disability, Chris was under tremendous stress. When a child psychiatrist "made him play school" with little toy people, he soon found out how frustrated Chris was. It also became clear that the rage attacks were not unprovoked, as previously thought, but were precipitated by seemingly minor unpleasant incidents. Analysis of the episodes showed that they were not temporal lobe seizures. The recognizing of Chris's learning disability led to more appropriate school management and within 2 months his temper tantrums disappeared.

Temporal lobe epilepsy very rarely presents itself in the form of an outburst of anger. These seizures are usually unprovoked and aimless. Such individuals are usually adolescents or young adults. They may realize that the attack is coming (aura) but are totally unaware of their irrational behavior during the seizure. The correct diagnosis (psychiatric or epileptic) is very delicate and difficult; however, it is obviously of great importance for appropriate management. Often a definite conclusion is reached only after elaborate and prolonged EEG studies that document the presence of electrical discharges during the attack.

Daydreaming

Everyone daydreams—apparently a necessary physiological phenomenon—but sometimes this can be excessive. Children who are bored, sleepy, tired, or preoccupied, just stare ahead for a few seconds or even minutes between their activities. The handicapped, the emotionally disturbed, or those with a disorder of attention tend to do it more commonly and for longer periods. When epilepsy is suspected, day dreaming may be mistaken for absence seizures (petit mal) or complex partial seizures (like temporal lobe epilepsy).

Staring due to daydreaming is not hard to identify because a tap on the shoulder or a little shake interrupt it at once, but do not usually stop a seizure. Children who daydream also blink to threat whereas those with absence seizures fail to do so. It is true that sometimes epileptic attacks may be so short that by the time the mother reaches the child they are over. Invariably, however, there are other subtle signs that indicate a seizure disorder. These may be a vacant look, slight twitching of the eyelids, rhythmic swallowing, fumbling, subtle confusion, or tiredness.

Tics and Jerks

Myoclonic seizures can sometimes be confused with nervous tics, repetitive habitual blinking, eyerolling, and jerky movements. Emotionally disturbed, mentally retarded, and autistic children may exhibit a set of bizarre movements. Myoclonic seizures are accompanied by electrical disturbances in the EEG, these tics, jerks, and bizarre movements are not. Therefore, close observation and an EEG clarify the diagnosis.

Fainting

Fainting is exceedingly common. Although it can occur at any age, fainting seems to be most frequent in later childhood and especially in girls during periods of active growth. It is occasionally mistaken for epilepsy. Typically these individuals are standing in a warm and perhaps stuffy atmosphere when they become pale, dizzy, and slowly slump to the ground. It may be seen with a rapid postural change to upright as when jumping out of bed in the morning. The cause of their "syncope" (fainting) is the diminished blood flow to the brain due to a fall in blood pressure. For this reason when the attack is coming, by lowering their heads between their knees, they prevent the fainting. On the ground the adequate blood flow returns to the brain and they become conscious again. Obviously, people rushing to the aid of these individuals should not pick them up but let them recover while lying flat. Headache or confusion are generally not present after the episode. Sometimes in more severe cases, associated jerking, stiffening of the body or incontinence of urine occur. A careful analysis of the circumstances in which the attacks happen allows a doctor to differentiate fainting from epilepsy.

Pallid Syncope (Reflex Vagal Syncope)

Ted Robinson, a 6-year-old, struck his head against the edge of a dinner table. He cried out, became very pale, and slowly slumped to the floor unconscious. He appeared to be lifeless but within 30 seconds, gradually some color appeared in his face and he woke up. He felt tired for the next hour but was all right afterward.

Mrs. Robinson took Ted to her family physician who referred him to a child neurologist. After obtaining a careful history, a type of fainting spell, called pallid or reflex vagal syncope, was diagnosed. During a subsequent EEG recording that was done with a simultaneous electrocardiogram, the doctor suddenly pressed on Ted's eyes. His heart immediately slowed down and actually stopped for several seconds. The child became very pale but as he was already lying down he did not faint. This test completed the diagnosis.

The doctor explained that sudden pain or anger, in some susceptible individuals, can trigger off a reflex which stops the heart for a very short time. A drop in blood pressure will cause dizziness and, if severe, a fainting. Mrs. Robinson was told that during such episodes she must never prop Ted up because then the blood flow to the brain would be further reduced. That, in turn, would not only prolong the spell but could even cause a convulsion. The doctor said Ted would outgrow his predisposition and that treatment was not necessary.

In susceptible children, often trivial but unexpected pain particularly to the head, fright, or other special stimulus such as sight of blood may precipitate a syncope. It can also be triggered for diagnostic purposes by applying sudden pressure on the child's eyes during an EEG or by reproducing in the lab the triggering stimulus such as showing "blood" (red paint on a piece of gauze). The underlying mechanism is not an emotional response but reflex inhibition, initiated by the nervous system upon the heart rate, which normally simply slows down. In oversensitive individuals such a reflex is excessive and the heart may stop for several seconds. Thereby the blood flow to the brain is drastically reduced and the child may feel dizzy then faint. When the episode is severe (keeping an individual upright makes it worse) convulsive movements could also occur. In such cases, the attacks closely mimic grand mal epilepsy. The heart rate soon becomes regular, the circulation resumes, and the child completely recovers although he or she may be tired for a while.

Individuals with this disorder tend to outgrow their predisposition. When the attacks are severe and frequent, continuous administration of atropine, which reduces this excessive reflex, can prevent their occurrences; otherwise treatment is not necessary. Anticonvulsant drugs are not helpful in this disorder. Understandably, misdiagnosis of epilepsy is harmful.

Breath-holding Spells

Breath-holding spells are common in early childhood. When susceptible children cry vigorously they may suddenly involuntarily catch their breath during expiration. Gradually their faces become blue because of the lack of oxygen and they fall back limp and unconscious. Occasionally there is an associated jerk or stiffening of the body and when this occurs, epilepsy may be diagnosed mistakenly. They soon recover and continue their activities as though nothing had happened.

The underlying mechanism is not fully understood. These spells cannot be prevented medically but they disappear spontaneously with age. The parents need to be assured about the benign nature of the attacks and should be warned not to overprotect their children.

Psychogenic Epilepsy

Psychogenic epileptic attacks (pseudo-seizures) are rare. Most are not difficult to diagnose by experienced neurologists. They may be a difficult problem if they occur, as sometimes they do, in people with true epileptic seizures. By having a "convulsion" just at the right time, in front of an audience, children occasionally recognize subconsciously that a seizure affects their parents or teachers. They learn that an attack may gain or avoid something. It may increase the attention their parents give them or deal with their worries about going to school. In other children, psychogenic epilepsy may represent a reaction to some underlying feelings. It may be because they are concerned about themselves or their families as for instance when they sense that the parents are having serious marital difficulties. Usually there is a dramatic, bizarre quality about these spells. They may start with a loud cry and be followed by falling, without injury, and "violent" thrashing around. Yet there is often remarkably quick recovery.

A 16-year-old girl who had been well-controlled on medications for several years began having a series of convulsions. The parents reported this to her physician who ordered an EEG and checked the blood levels of her medications. Since the convulsions seemed to be unusually strong and the tests were surprisingly good, the physician arranged an EEG with simultaneous video taping.

The waiting room at the hospital was full when the girl and her mother arrived. Soon after settling down she announced loudly that she was not feeling well and lay down on a bench. A few minutes later she suddenly groaned, then violently and rhythmically began to move her body up and down. She even used her arms to assist in the push. It was so dramatic that several people jumped up from their seats and ran for a doctor or a nurse.

During the EEG recording, as the physician looked on, he commented that it seemed as though another spell was developing. Within seconds the teenager's body was jerking up and down, but the EEG remained normal! With her "pseudo-seizures" the girl had fooled many people, including her parents. Later, a psychiatrist interviewed the family and with counseling these episodes disappeared.

Careful observations of pseudo-seizures usually reveals the correct diagnosis. Parents can perform a test by gently separating the person's eyelids; during a true seizure the eyes are usually open or the eyelids easily separate whereas in psychogenic epilepsy the "unconscious" person resists.

The development of pseudo-seizures, usually in teenagers or young adults whose epilepsy is otherwise under stable control, indicates that their emotional needs have not been met. It also means that their interpersonal relationships may be disturbed at a particularly delicate time when social and psychological demands are very stressful.

Psychogenic seizures present a medical condition just as serious as epilepsy although in a different way. These children should not be ridiculed or underestimated. Because of the many complex investigations required to establish the firm diagnosis, it is advisable to hospitalize them for a period of observation; it is unlikely that they will receive full consideration and support in any other setting. This is another example where a few days of intensive and well-coordinated teamwork between the neurologist, the nurses, the EEG technologists, the social workers, and the psychiatrist can be very rewarding. The understanding and cooperation of the parents, other family members and even the teachers is essential. The therapy, of course, is not to increase the anticonvulsants but to remove the causes of stress or improve the coping mechanisms.

chapter 7

What Parents Should Know about Treatment

How Drugs Work

How Medications Are Maintained

How Medications Are Started and Discontinued

Never Stop the Treatment on Your Own!

How Often Medications Need to Be Given

What If He Has Forgotten to Take His Pills?

Pills or Liquid?

Is My Child Going to Be an Addict?

Is an "Epileptic Always an Epileptic?"

What the Dentist Needs to Know

What Parents Need to Know about Pharmacies

Prescriptions

Why Parents Ask for a Second Medical Opinion

Both Parents Should Come for Appointments

How Drugs Work

After the diagnosis of epilepsy has been established, physicians begin to plan their treatment and they can choose from an increasing number of potentially effective drugs. The medications are selected for their ability to help prevent different types of seizures. This knowledge is based on animal studies and on previous experience with individuals who had epilepsy. Each child's situation may be slightly different, and the expected benefits of treatment may not immediately occur or troublesome side-effects could develop. A process of careful trial and error is necessary to determine which drug or combination is the most helpful. Medications are ordinarily given by mouth, although during emergencies intravenous, intramuscular and even rectal injections are used. The swallowed drug passes from the stomach to the small bowel where it is absorbed into the bloodstream. Here protein molecules carry it around. As the blood travels through the brain the drug diffuses into the liquid surrounding each nerve cell, and that is where the antiepileptic action occurs. When needed, intravenous administration of some anticonvulsants achieve a faster brain concentration.

The body continuously eliminates foreign substances. Most anticonvulsants, like other medications, are broken down by the liver and excreted by the kidneys, the complete elimination taking days, and even weeks. Prior to treatment, physicians screen the child's metabolism with blood tests because when it is abnormal serious side effects may develop. For example, when the liver or kidneys are not functioning well, the anticonvulsant blood levels can become very high, causing serious side effects. At times other medications may also interfere (anticonvulsants or not).

A young boy with epilepsy who was receiving Dilantin developed tuberculosis. Two weeks after the treatment for tuberculosis began he became increasingly lethargic. Naturally this caused great concern because it was feared that the disease not only affected the lungs but also the brain. The neurologist, however, found the Dilantin blood level to be markedly elevated. The antituberculosis medications interfered with the elimination of Dilantin and when the dosage was reduced the child's lethargy disappeared.

Another child was treated with phenobarbital but her epilepsy was not fully controlled. After Depakene was added the seizures stopped but she became increasingly drowsy and tired. Tests showed that the phenobarbital level was too high. Depakene slowed down the breakdown process of phenobarbital by the liver. After the dosage of phenobarbital was reduced the tiredness disappeared.

The same, or at times just the opposite, can occur with other drug combinations. For example, adding phenobarbital to Dilantin may increase its breakdown by the liver resulting in lower blood levels of Dilantin.

The exact mechanism of many anticonvulsants is not fully understood. It is beyond the scope of this book to try to describe the different hypotheses and findings in experimental studies. It will be sufficient to remember that medications, no matter how they work, do not cure epilepsy. They help the brain perform its functions by avoiding abnormal reactions—the seizures—but do not remove the cause of epilepsy, just as aspirin does not take away the cause of headaches.

How Medications Are Maintained

The daily "maintenance" dose is what the doctor recommends to be taken regularly in order to keep the amount of drug at sufficient levels all the time. The blood levels at which seizures are best controlled, with the least side effects, are known as the therapeutic range. The physician must prescribe just enough to balance the continuous elimination by the liver and kidneys. If the child takes more, the level in the blood will increase gradually until, as a result of this accumulation, signs of toxicity will develop. Therefore, for the side effects to become apparent it is not necessary to take an overdose. Toxicity may appear very slowly—even months after the last change in the dosage. Because of the subtle, gradual presentation, the real cause of the child's symptoms may be overlooked. Obtaining a blood level immediately, however, clarifies the situation. This issue is illustrated by the following case report and by Figure 1.

Roy, a 16-year-old, was taking 200 mgs. of Dilantin a day (A). The blood level was low so his physician increased the dose to 300 mgs. but this proved to be too much because the level rapidly increased beyond the

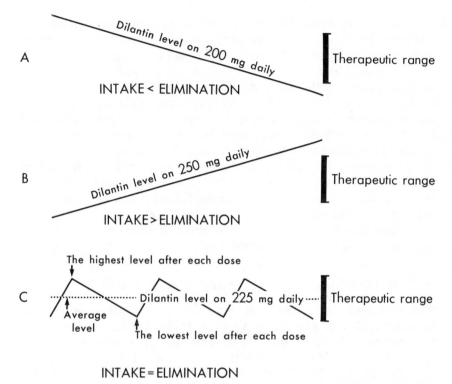

A Dilantin level on 200 mg daily   Therapeutic range
INTAKE < ELIMINATION

B Dilantin level on 250 mg daily   Therapeutic range
INTAKE > ELIMINATION

The highest level after each dose

C Dilantin level on 225 mg daily ···· Therapeutic range
Average level
The lowest level after each dose

INTAKE = ELIMINATION

Figure 1. This diagram shows how within the therapeutic range a satisfactory balance between drug intake and elimination was finally achieved by Roy's doctor.

therapeutic range. Then the doctor prescribed only 250 mgs. a day (B). Four weeks later the blood level was perfect but two months after this adjustment Roy became increasingly tired. His blood level was again above the therapeutic range; therefore, his physician reduced the dosage of Dilantin to 200 mgs. for 3 days, after which to 225 mgs. a day (C). Roy has been well since. Figure 1 explains this process.

Great progress has been made in the understanding of drug metabolism since the determination of blood levels became routinely available. The highest blood level occurs soon after the medication is administered and the lowest level before the next dose. The longer the interval between the doses the lower the level becomes. Obviously, this is also influenced by the rate at which drugs are metabolized and each drug is different. Some may be given once or twice a day and others four times. Whereas a doctor can easily suggest how frequently and how much medication to give, it is impossible to predict the way a person will absorb and then eliminate the drug from the body. This is an individual matter. There are ways to study these metabolic functions but they are cumbersome and expensive. So it is more practical to take an educated guess based on knowing how an average person with that body weight metabolizes that particular anticonvulsant. Then, a trial and error approach is used by observing the seizure control, watching for side effects and repeating blood levels. From the minimum of two blood levels taken at times when the child was on two different daily doses the desired amount of anticonvulsant can be calculated. This was exactly the information Roy's doctor was trying to extrapolate. Likewise, it can be estimated by observing changes in two subsequent blood levels without changing the dose. Unfortunately, the issue is often complicated by various other factors such as the interactions with other medications, just to mention the most common one.

How Medications Are Started and Discontinued

Although some anticonvulsants are effective soon after administration, it usually takes several days, even weeks, after the beginning of treatment until a stable blood level is reached. This is the reason, for example, why children with febrile seizures, who take phenobarbital only during a sudden febrile illness, are not protected against a convulsion.

When a new medication is given it is distributed in the brain, which is the main target, and in the body. Most anticonvulsants have a marked affinity for fatty tissues. While the brain is composed in large part of fatty substances, the drugs are also trapped by other fatty tissues in the body. Therefore, until the body stores are filled up, much useful medication is diverted away from the brain (Figure 2). As a consequence blood levels are slow to rise during the first few days if only a maintenance dose is prescribed from the beginning.

It is important that until the drug concentration in a child's body reaches a "steady state," blood levels are not conclusive. In Figure 1, A, B, and C represent "steady states" between input and output. Although the level of the drug continuously changes up and down in relation to the daily schedule of administration, the average level between fluctuations is represented by a steady line and, therefore, is predictable.

As discussed above, when therapy is started with a maintenance dose, during the first couple of weeks the medication circulat-

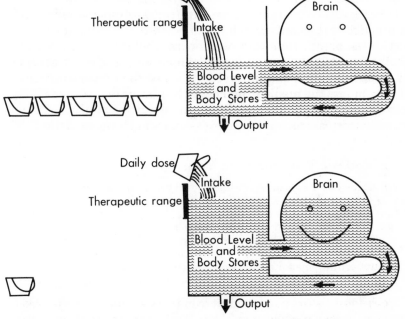

Figure 2.   When anticonvulsant therapy begins with maintenance doses, until the body stores are filled up much useful medication is diverted away from the brain. In case of emergency such a delay can be avoided by giving a large initial dose either orally or intravenously.

ing in the blood is not adequate for the brain. This is quite acceptable when there is no urgency in reaching the therapeutic level right away. In case of an emergency, however, such a delay can be avoided by giving a large initial dose either orally or intravenously. This is often successfully done with Dilantin. Most of the time, however, when at the start of treatment large amounts are prescribed (even maintenance) disturbing side effects may appear, such as dizziness, nausea, vomiting and lethargy. These are not due to excess medication but rather to an excessive response of the body to a foreign substance. It is wise, therefore, to give children time to adjust to a new drug gradually by starting with small doses and increasing them every so often. When side effects appear, the increments are slowed down or one or two doses are skipped. Usually with this careful method, anticonvulsants are built up to maintenance dose with a minimum of discomfort. It also gives the doctor a good estimate of the maximum daily medication an individual can tolerate.

When anticonvulsants are discontinued a slow depletion of body storage takes place, which will be reflected in a gradual decline of blood levels. Some drugs will fall more rapidly than others because of their faster metabolism and smaller body stores. If seizures recur, they happen as soon as the level falls below the therapeutic range and long before the medication is totally eliminated from the body. For this reason, most anticonvulsants have to be discontinued gradually, watching carefully for signs of seizures or changes in the EEG.

Never Stop the Treatment on Your Own!

John Howell was seizure-free for several years on phenobarbital. As he was 15 years old his parents allowed him to administer his own medication. Unexpectedly, he suffered a series of long, violent convulsions and had to be hospitalized. The seizures were controlled with intravenous medications but it was a frightening experience for everyone concerned. Surprisingly, John's initial blood test showed no detectable phenobarbital level. Later, he confessed to having stopped taking his pills a few days before because he thought it was no longer necessary.

Does John's story suggest that teenagers shouldn't be allowed to manage their own medications? Does it mean that parents need to be hovering in the background, looking over their shoulders to make sure a mistake is not made? This story should highlight the first five rules in the management of epilepsy, particularly communication. It is natural for one to become upset with being sick or having seizures and to wish for it to go away. It is understandable that children— even teenagers and adults—dream that if they didn't take medicine this would mean they weren't sick anymore. It is a dream, however, not reality.

Parents, their children and their physicians need to know and understand that these feelings are natural. There must be an atmosphere of trust and open communication about ideas so that they are not abruptly acted upon. There is nothing right or wrong about these feelings. People can make major mistakes, however, if they base their actions just on their emotions. Parents need to accept their children's feelings while continuing to discuss their understanding and knowledge with them and their doctors.

It is important to point out again that it takes only one or two days without medications to lower the blood level below the therapeutic range when problems may arise. The drug does not need to be completely eliminated from the body to cause major convulsions.

Nevertheless, as a rule anticonvulsants must be taken regularly as prescribed. When the treatment is gradually but prematurely discontinued, the seizures recur usually with their original pattern. When the treatment is abruptly stopped, however, the child may have dangerously violent recurrent and long convulsions called status epilepticus. These prolonged seizures are very difficult to treat and they can cause brain damage and even death. Parents, therefore, must never abruptly stop the medications without the doctor's knowledge! Physicians are careful when they stop antiepileptic medications. The lowering and discontinuation of most drugs must be gradual, sometimes spreading over several months.

How Often Medications Need to Be Given

Traditionally, anticonvulsants were given in three or four daily doses and exactly on time. With better understanding of drug metabolism, it became clear that most medications could be taken in just two doses, that is, in the morning and at night. Watching the clock is an unnecessary and undesirable burden on the family. A few drugs such as Depakene or Clonopin may still be recommended in three or four daily doses but children do not need to take their medications to school and should not be awakened during the night. The noon dose can easily be given in the early afternoon when the child returns from school. The night dose is commonly larger than the one in the morning and this results not only in less sedation during the day but better protection during the night and early morning.

As discussed above, drugs taken at regular intervals provide more constant blood levels. Excessive peaks in blood levels, during which side effects may become prominent, as well as excessive falls, during which the risk of having seizures is greater, must be avoided. Medication schedules should be tailored according to individual needs. Anticonvulsants are best taken after meals as they tend to irritate the inner lining of an empty stomach and consequently cause discomfort. The administration of medications should be a routine matter just like brushing teeth. Parents already know that helping their children establish good routines is a lot of work.

What If He Has Forgotten to Take His Pills?

George, a 16-year-old teenager, was taking his own Dilantin somewhat irregularly and without much parental supervision. After 3 days without any Dilantin, he became fearful about having seizures and to catch up, he swallowed a dozen capsules at one time. A few hours later, accompanied by his horrified mother, he staggered into the emergency ward, confused, unsteady, and tremulous. His Dilantin blood level had climbed far beyond the upper limit of the therapeutic range. His stomach was "washed out" and he was admitted to the hospital. His symptoms disappeared after a couple of days.

Even extra cautious parents or older children occasionally forget the medications. When a single pill is missed it may be given with the next dose (double dose). When a full day's dose is forgotten, it can still be taken the next day. This rule, however, cannot be taken indiscriminately because in dealing with certain drugs and large doses there is a real danger of intoxication. In addition, not all anticonvulsants carry the same risk of seizure relapse following a sudden drop in the blood level. Irregular administration of medications (poor compliance) is irresponsible because it commonly leads to seizures. It is difficult for physicians and others to help parents and children if the prescribed treatment is not followed faithfully. The family must develop a foolproof routine of their own that ensures that the drugs are taken regularly.

When a child is young the parents look after the medications but during the early teenage years this responsibility is gradually transferred. Initially, the parents may prepare the daily medication in little cups or they could collect a week's supply in one container. A good way to check how many times medication has been forgotten is by the number of pills remaining. They could also ask their pharmacist to organize the drugs in special packs although this is more expensive (Figures 3 and 4). Adolescents are often rebellious and may not take their pills regularly. Parents and older children in charge of their medications should clarify with their physicians the most appropriate plan of action in case of missing a dose. When in doubt they should always call their doctors.

Pills or Liquid?

Many children, often for psychological reasons, find it difficult to swallow pills or capsules and prefer liquid medications; these are generally more expensive. The prescription may direct: "Take one teaspoonful (5 ml) twice a day" but there are teaspoons of different sizes. One parent, after measuring the medications with a teaspoon for years, realized she had given only about half of the prescribed drug because her teaspoon was rather small. Parents could use small plastic measuring cups or syringes with which to squirt the accurate

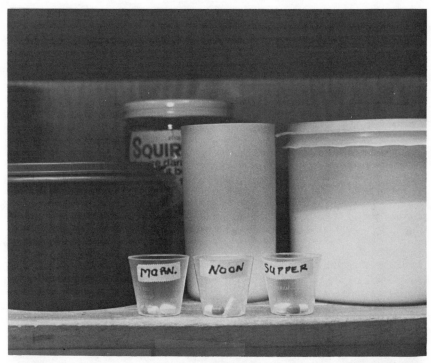

Figure 3.   During the early teenage years children should gradually assume responsibility for taking their own medications. Initially the parents may help by preparing the daily doses in small cups.

amount into the child's mouth. These cups or syringes should be rinsed after use (Figure 5).

Sometimes the prescription does not state the concentration of the liquid and physicians coming in contact with the child may not readily know the dosage. Concentrations often vary from one preparation to another. Most drugs are made of powder, which often does not dissolve in liquid. Liquid preparations of such medications are therefore "suspensions" in which the powder is simply mixed with a fluid vehicle. When the container is left unused for a while the powder tends to separate and to concentrate in the lower portion. Liquids and especially Dilantin suspensions, therefore, must be shaken thoroughly before use because the drug settles on the bottom of the container. Thus, without a good shaking, children initially receive less drug (during which period seizures may occur) whereas

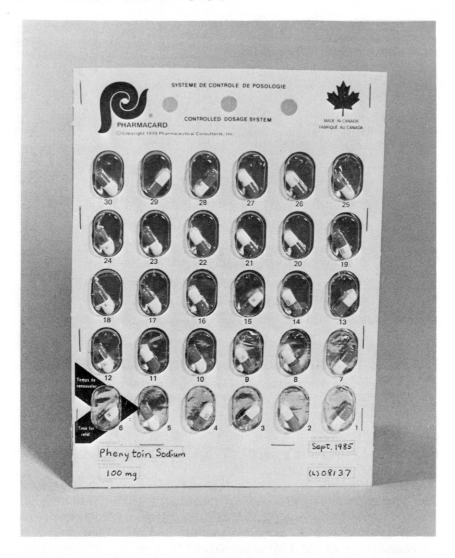

Figure 4. There are a variety of special packs that are helpful reminders for children to take their medications regularly. The pharmacist or the parent can fill them up for the month and then each day the drugs are removed.

later, as the suspension becomes more concentrated, they get too much (causing unwarranted side effects).

Liquid medications are not tasty even though they are prepared in sweet, flavored syrups. Many physicians prefer prescribing tab-

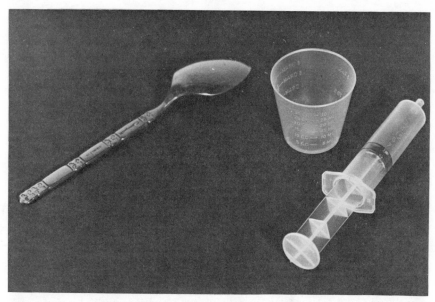

Figure 5. Administering liquid medications with teaspoons is less accurate than with measuring cups or syringes.

lets or capsules even to younger children because they can be accurately administered. Tablets can be cut in half or quarters when necessary and crushed. They can be given with jam, honey, or juice. Capsules can not be divided.

Most children do not enjoy taking their medicine and yet it is not necessary to convince them that they should like it. One can sympathize with their feelings but what is most important is that they learn the routine of taking their medicine and accepting it. After all, children don't need to like eating spinach or cleaning their own rooms—they need to learn to do it!

Is My Child Going to Be an Addict?

A young couple, who moved to a farm in order to escape city life and the drug culture, argued against the treatment of their infant with epilepsy. They could not see their daughter growing up "on drugs" especially since they were even avoiding aspirin and food additives. In their way of thinking, the occasional seizure was less harmful than the danger of "addiction."

Both the parental feelings of this sort and the rights of the child (a minor) to have the best possible treatment available, must be respected. The doctor has an important role in this arbitration. An objective discussion of the issues at stake will be helpful in reaching a reasonable decision.

It should be clear that anticonvulsants do not cause addiction as do the hard drugs, that is, cocaine, morphine, and heroin or relatively commonly used medication such as codeine, certain other pain killers, stimulants, and sleeping pills. Individuals with epilepsy do not take their treatment for pleasure or to get over an unpleasant problem, consequently they almost never abuse their medications. Studies have shown that there is no more danger of their becoming addicts than there is for any other person.

Pressure about whether to use treatment for epilepsy varies according to the type of seizures. Major convulsions are emotionally and socially detrimental and they do carry a definite risk for physical injury even if they are unlikely to cause brain damage. In such cases, a responsible doctor cannot accept fatalistic or distorted feelings of the parents and must protect the rights of the child by enforcing treatment. Physicians face similar moral obligations when parents, in good faith, refuse therapy for their child on the basis of religious beliefs; the physicians' arguments are less forceful when the child's attacks are infrequent and hardly noticeable because therapy does always carry the risk of side effects.

Doctors in general will favor treatment for two reasons: first, when the diagnosis of epilepsy, for example, petit mal or partial seizures, is firmly established, the possibility always exists that a generalized convulsion may occur even if it has never happened before; second, epileptiform electrical disturbances may be more frequent than suspected and may be accompanied by subtle cognitive and behavioral disturbances even if they do not cause overt seizures. Yet, there are few parents who, in view of very strong personal feelings, will still object to drugs. Because both views are valid, an acceptable compromise is to evaluate carefully the impact of EEG disturbance on the psychological (cognitive and emotional) functions before and after a period of treatment. Then a mutually acceptable decision may be reached in the best interests of the child.

While addiction to anticonvulsants does not occur, emotional dependence on treatment is common—understandably so—because having a seizure or witnessing it can be terrifying. Children sometimes "outgrow" their epileptic disorders so after several years of seizure-free periods physicians may try to discontinue the therapy. Most parents and children are delighted but some object and ask:

Shouldn't we just leave the medications the way they are? The discontinuation of therapy is based on the joint decisions of doctor, parents, and child.

Is an "Epileptic Always an Epileptic?"

It is difficult to generalize and to state how long children with epilepsy need to be treated because this depends on the type, onset, and severity of seizures, the response to drugs, on the EEG, age, and other variables. There are no foolproof rules and no absolute predictors to determine the possibility of relapse after the treatment is discontinued. Therefore, the issue of stopping medications should be openly discussed and carefully organized. Most doctors do not plan life-long therapy because, fortunately, many seizure disorders for little understood reasons spontaneously subside. This is especially true for the generalized epileptic attacks and more so for those without associated brain damage. Even children with severe disorders like infantile spasms and Lennox-Gastaut Syndrome may stop having seizures. In case of only one or rare convulsions in early childhood or certain types of partial seizures (for example Sylvian seizures) this is almost a certainty.

Children who have been seizure-free for a number of years and whose EEGs have returned to normal or almost so, may be allowed to discontinue their medications over several months. Physicians vary in their approaches, some being more and others less conservative but most are reluctant to stop treatment around puberty when significant hormonal changes occur, although scientific research does not support this. This is the age when a child who, for instance, has had absence seizures (petit mal) may start having generalized convulsions. On the other hand, after puberty and some time before the adolescents go for their driving licenses is a very appropriate time for finding out whether they still require therapy.

After the physician and the family have decided to stop the child's medications (it is perhaps best done during the summer to prevent the occurrence of seizures in school), there is also more time for electroencephalograms. If the attacks recur, treatment is usually restarted and it may be continued for another couple of years. When medications have controlled the seizures once, they will usually control them again. The fact that "an epileptic is not always an epileptic" is most important for the parents and the child to realize because hope can be very helpful in difficult situations. When the family knows that the eventual outcome may be good there is less anxiety and better adjustment. Every child with epilepsy is different, however, and unfortunately not all seizure disorders can be controlled. (The reader may notice that instead of *epileptic*, "the child with epilepsy" was used throughout the text. Many people feel that the word epileptic unnecessarily labels individuals.)

What the Dentist Needs to Know

The dentist should be informed when a child is being treated with Dilantin because it often produces marked and unsightly swelling (hypertrophy) of the gums (Figure 6). This predisposes a child to infection, therefore good dental care is important. Other anticonvulsants do not have this side effect.

Children on Dilantin must carefully brush and floss their teeth at least twice a day because good dental hygiene slows down and even prevents gum hypertrophy. Most children with thick gums have high Dilantin blood levels and merely adjusting the dose may help; otherwise, Dilantin needs to be replaced with another drug. As mentioned, excessive gum hypertrophy can be avoided but when it does occur dentists can resect a part of the excessively thickened gum in order to protect the child's teeth and to improve appearance. This, however, does not prevent further regrowth unless firm preventive measures are taken. Gum hypertrophy may represent a real problem when the child is mentally retarded, does not understand the importance of oral hygiene, and cannot cooperate.

What Parents Need to Know about Pharmacies

In many countries only physicians can order antiepileptic medications as these are strictly prescription drugs. Only the pharmacies originally providing the anticonvulsants may refill them and the prescription specifies how many times this can be done. Most doctors are willing to phone pharmacies for new prescriptions when requested to do so and if they are following the child regularly. Parents should be careful not to run out of medications on weekends when the regular pharmacy may be closed and/or the physician may be away. Because treatment should not be stopped under any circumstances, hospital emergency rooms may help to provide medications for 1 or 2 days.

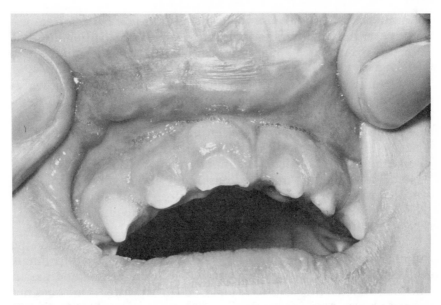

Figure 6. Dilantin therapy occasionally causes swelling of the gums. This complication can often be avoided.

Every prescription drug is known by brand (trade or proprietary) name and by generic (chemical) name. For example, Geigy produces Tegretol (brand) but the same substance is also known as carbamazepine (generic). Like other drugs certain anticonvulsants are produced by different manufacturers with competitive prices. Some anticonvulsants sold under their generic names are cheaper, yet most physicians prescribing them use the brand names because under the same generic name the medications, produced by a variety of manufacturers, may be slightly different. This might result in different absorption and in unwanted, and sometimes confusing, changes in blood levels, leading to seizure breakthrough. This has been noted with Dilantin and it may be true with Tegretol.

Drugs may cost more in one store than another so parents should shop around for the best deal. Because most anticonvulsants are stable products that do not lose their strength by aging, parents should not think that the lower price means that the drug might be spoiled. It is cheaper to buy larger quantities because the dispensing fee is the same for a small or large prescription. It is unwise to obtain a large supply, however, unless the treatment is well-established.

Pharmacies do not take medications back. Some pharmacists are more careful than others in explaining the administration and side effects of drugs; this should influence parents when deciding where to buy.

Occasionally Medicare, Medicaid, Pharmacare, or other health insurance or state programs pay for the prescription drugs. The family can inquire about eligibility from a social worker or a nurse at the hospital or clinic where they are obtaining medical care. When these resources are not available and if the prescription is sizable (at least 6 months supply) anticonvulsants can be obtained from the Epilepsy Foundation of America Pharmacy Service at a significantly cheaper rate. For prompt service the letter should be addressed to: E.F.A. Pharmacy Service, 126 South York Road, Hatboro, Pa., U.S.A. 19040.

It is requested that the original prescription, indicating the number of refills, should be sent. The bill, plus the cost of postage, will be included in the package received. The name and address on the back of each prescription must be clearly printed. One does not have to be an American citizen or a member of the Foundation in order to receive drugs. This pharmacy also stocks other medications.

Prescriptions

Almost everybody has heard a joke about the handwriting of physicians. In addition, prescriptions are written out with abbreviations and symbols. The deciphering is done by pharmacists who give careful and understandable directions on the bottle. Nevertheless, there are times when parents receive reports, notes, or directions directly from their physicians, which may or may not be seen by the pharmacists. Parents should be certain they understand their doctor's prescription. Another source of confusion is the strength of the medication prescribed. Although by regulations the name and strength of the drug must be written on the container, it is desirable for the parents to understand that information clearly before they leave their doctor's office. What they were told and what is written on the bottle should be the same; otherwise, they should call their physician at once.

A neurosurgeon who had just discharged Richard from the hospital carefully and conscientiously discussed his impressions with the parents. He mentioned that Richard should take his medications BID (meaning twice a day)—a common term used by doctors. The mother incorrectly assumed that BID meant once a day so she reduced her son's medications by one-half. Five days later, after an unexpected shower of seizures, the mistake was discovered.

Some of the commonly used Latin prescription abbreviations are shown in Table 1.

Why Parents Ask for a Second Medical Opinion

The sadness and dismay aroused after hearing that their child has epilepsy leads some parents to search for a different diagnosis. Seeing another physician can also keep alive the hope for a cure. Second opinions are commonly resorted to when the seizure control is poor, the child seems overmedicated, or when the family fails to understand the nature of the problem. At times a second opinion helps reconcile parents to accepting and not denying that there is a long-term medical disorder. It can confirm and clarify the diagnosis, as well as give rise to a new sense of direction and more effective treatment.

Who the best physician is in treating a child with epilepsy is discussed in Chapter 2. How to go about finding an expert second opinion may be difficult and confusing. Many factors are involved, such as the attending physician's reaction to the request, the availability of specialists, where the family is living and even their financial situation. It is probably most advantageous to find a neurologist who has experience with both children and seizures. When a child

Table 1. Commonly Used Latin Prescription Abbreviations

Abbreviations	Translations
po	Orally
ac	Before meals
pc	After meals
lc	Between meals
qd	Daily
BID	Twice daily
TID	Three times daily
QID	Four times daily
q6h	Every six hours
prn	As often as necessary
Stat	At once
ad lib	At pleasure (when one feels like it)

with epilepsy has other handicaps a multidisciplinary team approach may be the most helpful (see Chapter 13).

When parents are thinking about obtaining another medical opinion they should openly discuss their reasons with the attending physician. Local epilepsy societies and families of other children with seizure disorders can also be very informative. Parents should recall some of the basic rules that have been emphasized throughout this book: collaboration, trust, understanding, knowledge, communication, and also to use other sources of information.

Both Parents Should Come for Appointments

Whenever possible, both parents should come with their child to office or clinic visits. This is especially important at the time of diagnosis and in the early stages of treatment.

> Anna Cook, a toddler, developed frequent seizures. The mother became so preoccupied with her only child's care that her marriage began to take second place. Anna's father was also genuinely concerned but because of his job commitments he did not accompany his wife to office visits. In fact, he seemed to withdraw himself from his child's medical problems and let his wife shoulder the responsibilities; both parents were upset, afraid, angry, and tense.
>
> Just a few months ago, Mr. and Mrs. Cook's social life was flourishing; now it was ruined. Also, until recently Mr. Cook had been receiving much more attention so he felt his wife had lost interest in him. He did not fully realize the enormous pressures his wife was under, and Mrs. Cook became resentful because her husband did not help. Gradually, the marriage grew cool and so strained that they were ready to break up.
>
> During an office visit Mrs. Cook tearfully mentioned her strained marriage and said that "her husband doesn't seem to care" about Anna. When he heard this the physician insisted that, in spite of his busy schedule, Mr. Cook should come in for the next appointment. When they were both present the physician explained that at times like this because parents love their children they are scared, anxious, and even angry. They may become so preoccupied with the medical problem that they tend to neglect one another. He stressed that parents must communicate their feelings during these difficult periods and that both should come for office visits. Together, they must shoulder major health problems such as Anna's.
>
> Anna's seizures were eventually reasonably well-controlled. Now, whenever possible, both parents come to the office and they have dealt with their marital problems."

Parents can be so upset during the initial office visit that they may not remember much about the discussion with their doctor.

When only one parent is present it could be difficult to accurately answer all the questions that the absent spouse may ask. In such circumstances the parent can ask for a copy of the medical report; some even ask if they may tape record their conversation with the health professional. While these ideas are helpful, parents together, from the start, must share all the responsibilities of raising their child with epilepsy.

chapter 8

What Parents Should Know about Medications

Selection of Medications

Side Effects

Measurements: Weight, Volume, and Length

Common Drugs and Their Side Effects

Where Should the Medication Be Kept?

When Medical Treatment Fails

Quack Advice

Protective Helmets

What to Do for Accidental Overdosage

How to Give Medications to an Uncooperative Child

Selection of Medications

Physicians who treat epilepsy nowadays find themselves in a more favorable position than their colleagues 30 to 40 years ago because they can choose from an increasing number of drugs. The selection of medications depends first of all on the type of epilepsy, then on age and health, frequency and severity of seizures, response, side effects, and the physician's familiarity with the latest therapy.

The treatment usually begins with one drug, rarely two. Occasionally, a large initial loading dose is prescribed, especially when there are frequent seizures. During the next few weeks the daily dosage is adjusted according to the blood level of the anticonvulsant and the child is carefully watched. As discussed in Chapter 7, many of the anticonvulsants do not exert their full effect until after 2 or 3 weeks; therefore, premature changes or early conclusions about their ineffectiveness are unwise. Not infrequently, a drug trial (adequate blood levels for 3 or 4 weeks of duration) that fails with one child will be successful with another. Even though there are general guidelines, unfortunately the only way to find out for sure whether a drug is helpful is to try it. Trials are lengthy because medications often have to be increased slowly, step by step, in order to avoid undue reactions and to monitor carefully and systematically the effect on seizure frequency. Despite these precautions, they are often frustrating because side effects may appear before the control of epilepsy is achieved, requiring withdrawal of the drug. This process becomes even more complicated when children have more than one type of seizure because they will likely need a combination of medications.

Side Effects

All drugs, even the simplest ones such as aspirin, have potential side effects. Therefore, the risk is lower when the seizures can be controlled with one medication rather than two or more. At the time a drug is introduced, parents should expect to be told about possible adverse reactions. The pharmacist, when filling out a prescription, can also provide helpful information.

Side effects are the undesirable consequences of medications. They can be classified into two main groups. One is commonly seen, dose-dependent, and predictable while the other is rare, unrelated to the dose, totally unexpected and is due to individual predisposition and perhaps environmental conditions. The first type consists of subjective complaints (symptoms) such as dizziness, double vision, nausea, lethargy, irritability, unsteadiness, fatigue, weakness, poor appetite, and signs like increased hair growth or temporary loss of hair, thickening of the gums. These side effects are usually proportional to the dose. They are predictable because they are related to the nature of the medication (a sedative or stimulant), to the body parts affected (as for example brain or muscle) and to the organs through which the drugs are eliminated (kidney, liver). Sooner or later most people on treatment will experience these side effects according to their own individual tolerance, which varies from person to person. They disappear after decreasing the dosage or discontinuing the therapy. If tolerance for one medication is high the chances are greater that the doses could be taken in sufficient amount to control the seizures. But if the tolerance is low sometimes physicians and the parents may even wonder which is worse—the seizures or the treatment. When a child is seizure-free but winds up sleeping all the time or is unable to think because of overmedication, that treatment is not worthwhile. Parents should inquire about the drugs prescribed to their child so they know exactly what to expect.

Allergic reactions to specific medications belong to the second group. These could affect the bone marrow, liver, kidney, skin, and other parts of the body. To detect them, physicians check periodically the blood cell count, liver enzymes, and urine in most individuals on anticonvulsant treatment. Allergic reactions usually occur after a short period of therapy, often within the first 2 weeks. Most often it is a skin rash that can be mild to severe. It frequently spreads all over the body and it is very itchy but as soon as the drug is discontinued the skin clears up. On rare occasions the rash is so severe that hospitalization and special treatment is required. Once the medication is discontinued it cannot be started again without the risk of an even more severe allergic reaction. Fortunately in most instances the rash is coincidental and is due to a viral infection, other type of allergy, or irritation. For instance, when the rash appears long after the drug was started (several weeks or months) it is generally due to something else.

The physician must be absolutely sure that the rash was caused by a particular anticonvulsant before eliminating it from the treatment. If the rash is mild, the doctor may lower the dose and treat the child for a while with antihistamines (medications used for treating allergies). Slight drug reactions are often transient and benign so the therapy may be continued in full once the body has adjusted. Occasionally if it is essential, reintroduction of a medication that has caused a more severe rash in the past, may be attempted. This should be done with great caution and under the direct supervision of the physician. It must be understood that as in the cases of other drugs, such as aspirin or penicillin, allergic reactions to anticonvulsants are unpredictable.

Parents can report the side effects belonging to the first group during their next visit or sooner according to the severity. The physician, however, must be notified immediately when allergic reactions related to current treatment occur.

Measurements: Weight, Volume, and Length

Parents who are familiar with grains, pounds, ounces, pints, inches, and feet, are often mystified by the metric system, which is now universally used in medicine. In children, the total daily dose of an anticonvulsant is usually calculated on the basis of body weight in kilograms (kg) and it is written on the prescription in grams (gm) or milligrams (mg). Liquid medications are prescribed in milliliter (ml) or cubic centimeter (cc) and the child's height or size are measured in centimeters (cm). Table 1 shows the basic units of the metric system and Table 2 gives the conversions.

Table 1. Basic units of the metric system

Units	Metric System
Weight	1 gram (gm) = 1000 milligrams (mg)
	1 kilogram (kg) = 1000 grams
Volume	1 litre (L) = 1000 milliliter (ml, cc)
Length	1 centimeter (cm) = 10 millimeter (mm)
	1 meter (m) = 100 centimeter (cm)

Table 2.   Conversion table

Unit	Conversion
Weight	64.8 mg = 1 grain
	1 gm = 15.4 grains
	0.45 kg = 1 pound
	1 kg = 2.2 pounds
Volume	28.41 ml = 1 fluid ounce
	1 L = 35.2 fluid ounces
	1 cm = 0.39 inches
Length	2.54 cm = 1 inch
	30.48 cm = 1 foot
	1 m = 3.28 feet

Common Drugs and Their Side Effects

All antiepileptic drugs are known by their trade or brand name and also by their generic or nonproprietary names. Table 3 lists the more commonly used medications and their indications.

Every drug has potential side effects but most can be avoided or minimized when the physician and the parents carefully observe the child, and adjust the dosage according to the blood levels and to tolerance. The guideline in selecting the medications and dosage for long-term treatment is to use the drugs that offer the best seizure control with the least untoward effects. Table 4 shows some of the more common possible side effects.

The following case histories and drug reviews will illustrate some of the more common complications arising from treatment.

The Hydantoins

After a routine office visit, Mrs. Lewis mistakenly doubled the daily dose of Dilantin, which her step-daughter, Linda, was taking. Four to five days later Linda began complaining of dizziness, tiredness, and unsteadiness. She was excessively drowsy and could not concentrate in school. Mrs. Lewis promptly arranged a clinic visit.

Linda's neurological examination revealed jerky eye movements (nystagmus), particularly when she looked to either side. Her reach was tremulous and she was unsteady when walking (ataxia). These findings suggested Dilantin overdosage. A blood test was ordered and the Dilantin level was high. After stopping the medication for 2 days, since the above complaints disappeared, the blood level returned to normal. The drug was restarted in more appropriate dosage. After this episode,

Table 3.   Commonly used antiepileptic drugs

Trade, Brand Name(s)	Generic, Nonproprietary
Celontin	methsuximide
Clonopin (Rivotril in Canada)	clonazepam
Depakene	valproic acid
Diamox	acetazolamide
Dilantin	phenytoin
Luminal	phenobarbital
Mebaral	mephobarbital
Mesantoin	mephenytoin
Milontin	phensuximide
Mogadon	nitrazepam
Mysoline	primidone
Paradione	paramethadione
Tegretol	carbamezepine
Tranxene	clorazepate
Tridione (Trimedone in Canada)	trimethadione
Valium	diazepam
Zarontin	ethosuximide

each time Mrs. Lewis visited the clinic, she asked her doctor to write down the medications for her on a sheet of paper.

When Dilantin is taken on an empty stomach, it may cause some discomfort so it is best given with meals. The early signs of overdosage are persistent or intermittent double or blurred vision, drowsiness, unsteadiness, and tremulousness. These conditions all disappear as soon as the dosage is adjusted. Common side effects from long-term treatment, especially in children, are the gradual thickening of the gum (gum hypertrophy or hyperplasia) (Figure 6, Chapter 7), and excessive body hair growth (hirsutism). Both complications are cosmetically undesirable but not dangerous. Unlike gum hyperplasia, excessive hair remains on the body after the drug is discontinued. It can be removed by electrolysis. Excessive gum tissue can be resected surgically if it interferes with chewing or is too disfiguring. This side effect of Dilantin, at least in part, can be prevented by careful dental hygiene. In adolescents, who are already prone to acne, Dilantin may make the skin eruptions much more severe. To some extent the skin and the bone may also become thicker. See Chapter 7 for more information on Dilantin.

Table 4. Possible side effects of antiepileptic drugs

Drug	Side Effect
Celontin	Stomach upset, tiredness, dizziness, headache, rash*.
Clonopin (Rivotril)	Drowsiness, unsteadiness, tiredness, drooling.
Depakene	Weight gain, stomach upset, changes in liver function*.
Diamox	Drowsiness, dizziness, tiredness, rash*.
Dilantin	Stomach upset, jerky eye movements, poor balance, double vision, drowsiness, gum hypertrophy, overgrowth of hair, severe acne, rash*.
Luminal (phenobarbital)	Drowsiness, hyperactivity*, tiredness, rash.
Mebaral	Similar to Luminal, but less hyperactivity.
Mesantoin	Similar to Dilantin, bone marrow depression.
Milontin	Similar to Celontin.
Mogadon	Similar to Clonopin.
Mysoline	Similar to Luminal.
Paradione	Stomach upset, drowsiness, visual disturbance, rash*, low blood count* and kidney disturbance*.
Tegretol	Drowsiness, trouble focusing, rash*, low blood count*.
Tranxene	Similar to Clonopin
Tridione	Similar to Paradione but more visual disturbance (glare) and hiccup*.
Valium	Drowsiness, unsteadiness, tiredness.
Zarontin	Stomach upset, tiredness, dizziness, headache, rash*.

*If severe, it usually requires immediate withdrawal of the medication. All side effects should be brought to the attention of the physician.

Mesantoin, which is rarely used, is similar to Dilantin. It does not cause thickening of the gum but there is a higher risk of bone marrow depression.

The Barbiturates

There are three commonly used barbiturates: phenobarbital, Mebaral, and Mysoline. The phenobarbital has been used in the treatment of epilepsy for 70 years while the other two were introduced 30 to 40 years ago. Their action and side effects are somewhat similar: drowsiness, dizziness, tiredness, and hyperactivity.

Robert's seizures responded well to phenobarbital but his behavior changed dramatically. Robert, who was 3 years old, almost overnight became cranky and tired but he still had inexhaustible energy. His attention seemed to shift rapidly from one toy to another, he was always in a hurry—to the point of tripping over things and bumping into objects. He could not relax, had great difficulty falling asleep and awakened frequently. After a couple of weeks, the tired parents were ready to give up. Fortunately, phenobarbital could be replaced with another anticonvulsant and within a couple of days Robert was a pleasant boy again.

Hyperactivity, resulting from phenobarbital treatment is a common paradoxical reaction in children, and it should not be ignored when it occurs even to a slight degree. Reducing the dosage is rarely beneficial; substituting Mebaral for phenobarbital may occasionally help but most of the time a new anticonvulsant needs to be started.

Mysoline is the most recently introduced barbiturate. In the body it is broken down to a compound that is effective as an anticonvulsant and also to phenobarbital. Naturally, additional phenobarbital therapy should not be given when Mysoline is prescribed. The drug should be started in small doses and built up gradually in order to avoid a variety of side effects at the beginning of treatment.

Carbamezepine

Tegretol is a relatively new and very effective anticonvulsant medication with only a few side effects. It has become one of the most commonly used drugs in the treatment of epilepsy.

> Elizabeth was 10 years old when she was diagnosed as having temporal lobe epilepsy. Tegretol, now considered the drug of choice in complex partial seizures (temporal lobe epilepsy) was selected and the young girl was immediately placed on full daily doses. She became dizzy and very tired. The parents were so concerned that they requested their physician to review the treatment. He assured them that this was a transient side effect.

Tegretol may occasionally cause drowsiness and tiredness during the initial 2 to 3 weeks of treatment, mainly when full doses are started at once. When the initial dosage is moderated, side effects are minimal and subside early. Therefore, most physicians prefer to build up the dose of Tegretol gradually in order to minimize the initial sedation. The barbiturates or other drugs like Valium or Clonopin may even be worse in this respect and require a very slow increase.

Some adolescents and occasionally younger observant children may complain of difficulty in focusing their eyes on a target. This is not quite the same as the "double vision" described with Dilantin treatment. This disturbance is intermittent; it is most bothersome within 1–2 hours after taking each dose. It can be minimized by giving a larger portion of Tegretol at bedtime and smaller doses during the day. In this way the medication in the daytime is better tolerated without loss of effectiveness because the total daily medication is unchanged.

The physician will always require a complete blood count as a baseline before starting Tegretol because a slow-down in the production of white blood cells in the bone marrow is to be expected. The normal white blood count is at around 6–7000/mm3. Lower counts are well tolerated but when they reach 2000/mm3 then the child's resistance to bacterial infections may be diminished. This depression of bone marrow activity occurs within the first 6 months of treatment. Lowering the dosage temporarily usually helps. Later, the occasional diminished blood count is most likely related to viral infections (such as a cold or flu-like illnesses). In any case the blood test should be repeated within a week and no changes in dosage are necessary if the count has returned to baseline.

Tegretol is particularly well tolerated by youngsters. It is remarkably free of adverse behavioral side effects—so frequently encountered when for instance phenobarbital is used in this age group. Parents commonly comment that their child's behavior was better after the treatment with Tegretol began.

Valproic Acid

Depakene has only recently been introduced in North America. It is especially useful in treating absence spells (petit mal), myoclonic seizures, primary generalized convulsions (grand mal) and even other types of epilepsy. Depakene might affect the liver enzymes, therefore, tests need to be done repeatedly. If affected, lowering the daily dose usually helps and there is no need to switch to another medication. On extremely rare occasions and only in very young children rapid fatal liver illness occurs, which is due to a catastrophic allergic reaction. Most children on this treatment are alert and their appetites are good; in fact, weight gain may be a problem. Nausea and loss of appetite are not infrequent side effects particularly in the early weeks of treatment. They can be avoided when the drug is taken with meals, the same daily medication is given more frequently or if the dose is lowered slightly. Children on Depakene who will be having surgery should have their bleeding and clotting time checked because it could be abnormal.

The Succinimides

Zarontin is another important anticonvulsant. It is useful in the treatment of absence spells (petit mal) and to a lesser extent for myoclonic seizures. One of its advantages is that it does not sedate and unlike Depakene, it is not offensive to the liver. Milontin and Celontin are closely related to Zarontin. They are less commonly prescribed because of their potential adverse reactions, but they are also less effective.

In some individuals Zarontin may cause unpleasant stomach upset (heart burn, nausea, loss of appetite). These complaints are noted mainly at the onset of therapy and when the capsule form is used. The drug is better tolerated after meals and especially when the syrup or elixir form is prescribed. In certain cases an antacid may help. If all these measures do not alleviate the stomach upset even though the medication controls the seizures, as a last resort Zarontin could be replaced by Celontin, which may be equally effective. These two drugs are marketed in relatively large capsules. For those who find them difficult to swallow a liquid form is available. One teaspoonful of medicine is the same as a capsule. Parents should be reminded again that there are varying sizes of teaspoons and for measuring purposes a teaspoon should contain 5 ml of liquid. Pharmacists will provide measuring cups or syringes on request.

The Diazepines

Valium is primarily a tranquilizer and a muscle relaxant, so it is not surprising that when it is used as an anticonvulsant the main side effect is excessive sedation. Valium is a powerful, rapidly acting antiepileptic drug that is most effective when administered intravenously or more recently, rectally. Because it can quickly stop convulsions it is of great use in the emergency rooms. The effect of Valium is short lived, therefore repeated intravenous injections at frequent intervals may be required. This should be done under direct medical supervision because it not only stops seizures but can also depress other vital functions such as respiration. This is especially so if the individual is already receiving other anticonvulsants particularly phenobarbital. Due to the slow absorption, Valium given by mouth is more effective for anxiety than seizures.

Clonopin (Rivotril in Canada), which was recently introduced, belongs to the same group of drugs as Valium. It is more effective orally than Valium and it is used in the treatment of many epileptic disorders particularly myoclonic seizures and infantile spasms. Its major side effect is sedation, therefore it should be administered in small doses several times a day. Occasionally young children drool and seem mucousy while taking it. This constitutes a considerable limiting factor in mentally retarded children who already have a tendency to drool profusely. Often Clonopin controls seizures for several months but then due to seizure breakthrough, the dose has to be increased to the point where the child may become over sedated.

Tranxene and Mogadon are the most recently introduced diazepines. Their action and side effects are similar to those of Clonopin.

Other Drugs

Diamox is primarily a diuretic but at times is dramatically effective in the treatment of petit mal. It is best administered three to four times a day. Although it may increase drinking to compensate for the greater urine output, it is virtually free of serious side effects. Some individuals, however, may experience drowsiness.

The "diones" (paradione and Tridione) are old and are replaced by a new generation of drugs. They are effective against absence spells (petit mal) and even tonic-clonic convulsions (grand mal). They are still used occasionally when other anticonvulsants have failed.

Where Should the Medication Be Kept?

Antiepileptic medications are best kept in tightly closed, child proof containers, in a dry cool place, away from heat or direct sunlight and not in the bathroom where humidity is high. They should never be placed in a freezer. Left over drugs are a constant hazard for small children and some may become toxic in time. As a rule, when medications are no longer needed they should be discarded unless otherwise specified by the physician. When doing so, throw it in the toilet and not in the garbage, which is often accessible to small children or pets.

When Medical Treatment Fails

There are some children whose seizures cannot be stopped by medications in spite of repeated investigations, consultations, and many different drug trials. This can be an extraordinarily stressful time for both the children and their families—the stress not only making it more difficult for everyone but perhaps also creating further problems. Many people feel they can handle things alone as they do not wish to depend on others, but talking to someone else and especially a person who understands can be very helpful at this time. Therefore, when the physician suggests a referral to a social worker, psychologist, or psychiatrist, neither the parents nor the child should view themselves as persons with emotional disorders.

Special diets containing an excess of fat (ketogenic diet) are occasionally used for myoclonic seizures that have not responded to other more conventional treatments. As the fat is digested, the blood becomes more acidic than normal and may diminish or entirely stop the seizures. This diet can only be given under the careful supervision of a qualified dietitian and the physician. Unfortunately, the diet is not a tasty one and requires much work on the part of the parents.

> Frank Kelly, a 7-year-old, had poorly controlled epilepsy, cerebral palsy and moderate mental retardation. He was attending a special class for slow children and had to wear a helmet for protection. Since the age of 2 years, with not much success he was treated with a combination of anticonvulsants for his frequent drop attacks, myoclonic jerks and major convulsions.
>
> As the last resort it was decided to try ketogenic diet. Frank was admitted to the hospital and for the first 2 days he was observed and a number of basic tests were done while he was fasting. When the urine began to show ketones (a breakdown product of fatty tissue) the special diet was started. It was very high in fatty foods and low in carbohydrates. Although the meals were not tasty Frank cooperated. His stools became bulky and sometimes liquid but his seizures dramatically subsided. Later some of the anticonvulsants were discontinued and Frank was much more alert in school. The parents were pleased with the treatment even though this meticulous diet was time-consuming for Mrs. Kelly.

Often in the past the ketogenic diet had to be discontinued because the children refused to eat it. With the introduction of MCT oil (medium chain trygliceride) the diet is better tolerated and parents do not need to be so terribly restrictive with candies, bread, and other carbohydrates. The MCT oil is a synthetic compound that is tasteless and can replace fatty foods such as butter, corn oil, and bacon. Strict discipline, however, is still required, which affects the whole family. It may be troublesome when the child does not understand, is not cooperative, and when other young children are around. Craving for sweets can be so great that the food has to be kept locked up. Adequate vitamin intake should be maintained, the parents need to check the urine daily, and must review the diet periodically with the dietitian, the clinic nurse, or the physician. Because of the strain involved, the ketogenic diet should be the last resort in the treatment of intractable seizure disorders. In certain cases it can be extremely effective and beneficial especially in the age group before puberty. If well-conducted it does not prevent normal growth, does not lead to obesity or to metabolic diseases. The long-term consequences, however, of high blood fat content on the arteries, heart, liver, and other organs is unknown. For this reason it is advisable to discontinue the diet after several months and restart it only if deemed absolutely necessary.

Surgery is another possible answer for a restricted number of children with epilepsy.

> Julie McNaulty was 16 months old when she was involved in a car accident. Investigations in the hospital revealed a right-sided skull fracture with a large collection of blood underneath; this was immediately drained by a neurosurgeon but the right side of the brain was severely damaged. Ever since the accident, in spite of heavy medication, Julie had been having seizures—even several hundred times a day. Her development slowed down and gradually she began to regress. Repeated CAT scans confirmed that the damage was on the right side of the brain only and a series of EEGs showed the seizures to be originating also from that side, particularly from one area. It was proposed to the parents that the damaged part of the brain be removed in order to stop the seizures. Julie was thoroughly investigated by a team of physicians and psychologists. A psychiatrist and a social worker dealt with the family and a final decision was reached in favor of surgery. The operation lasted for 6 hours. Julie's seizure control improved dramatically and her development began to improve.

Neurosurgery is only considered as a form of treatment when it is firmly established that the epilepsy cannot be controlled by medications. Also the seizures must come mainly from one area of the brain (which can be safely removed) and be so frequent that they prevent the child from having a reasonably normal life.

In recent years revolutionary new neuroradiological techniques were developed such as radioactive and CAT scanning of the brain. They can now be used routinely along with EEGs. Not infrequently, after years of seizures believed to be idiopathic in origin, a lesion is discovered by these tests. This is occasionally a slow growing tumor that all along has been responsible for the epilepsy. In such cases surgery becomes a primary consideration. The aim in surgery for epilepsy is the radical removal of the underlying lesion that causes the seizures, with minimal sacrifice of healthy brain tissue. Although some loss of function is to be expected after such an operation, on the long range it can be adequately compensated. In addition, it must be understood that certain parts of the brain can not be operated upon because they are too close to areas controlling essential functions (speech, memory, etc.), the loss of which would be more devastating than epilepsy itself. It is beyond the scope of this book to discuss the complex and careful investigations necessary to decide whether a surgical intervention can be of real benefit to the child. Parents should know that this issue can be discussed with their doctor at any time. They should also realize that specialized centers exist where all appropriate tests (including detailed neuro-psychological and psychiatric evaluations) can be performed. Naturally, the thought of brain surgery is frightening for anyone. In certain emergency situations, however, it is lifesaving and can also be quite successful in controlling different forms of epilepsy. In carefully selected individuals it has improved considerably the quality of life.

Unfortunately when the whole brain is involved at once as in the generalized epilepsies or when the responsible lesion can not be identified, surgery is not indicated.

Behavioral treatment approaches are occasionally employed in the management of epilepsy by using reward and punishment, self-control, and other psycho-physiological techniques. Children who, in spite of medication, still have many and severely disrupting seizures and who are not candidates for diets or surgery, may benefit from this type of approach.

> Rose Kaplan was a 17-year-old mentally retarded girl with drop seizures. She was maintained quite satisfactorily on medications until she began her overbreathing episodes. It is difficult to say why she picked up this self-stimulating behavior of repeatedly deep breathing for 5 to 15 minutes at a time, 20 to 30 times a day. Her overbreathing frequently precipitated a seizure which caused her to crash to the floor or against the furniture. Since Rose just would not listen to reasoning, the parents, teachers, nurses, counselors, and physicians were at a complete loss. Finally a psychologist, who was familiar with epilepsy, was consulted and she recommended placing smelling salts under the girl's nose each time she began to overbreath. This had a dramatic effect on her. Rose no longer found overbreathing pleasurable and the episodes stopped.

Identifying and removing external or internal factors that precipitate seizures represents a rational form of prevention. Behavior modification techniques include also a number of self-control procedures to diminish physical and emotional stress so often related to the presence of seizures. This task is accomplished through a meticulous account being kept over a long period of time of the circumstances under which the attacks occurred. The key to success and prevention is the identification of all possible precipitating factors.

This requires considerable insight on the part of the child with epilepsy, and the parents in addition to expert counseling. An additional benefit is that increased self-awareness prevents excessive dependence on medications and leads to a more structured, better organized life style.

Quack Advice

Families of children with epilepsy frequently receive from relatives and friends advice that is not always helpful. A common suggestion is that they see another doctor or that they travel to a well-known medical center. Indeed, occasionally there is a need for additional opinions but this should be openly discussed with the child's physician: failure to do so could lead to a disturbed relationship and/or to unnecessary financial burdens for the family.

Parents, from the most naive to the best informed, are strongly motivated to help their children. In searching for the "best" they sometimes can be taken advantage of by people looking for an easy income.

> A well-mannered, professional-looking quack "doctor" promised the parents that if they would carry out his recommendations, he would cure their child of epilepsy. The anticonvulsants were abruptly discontinued and the child was given only salad and goat's milk. It is difficult to believe that the parents followed such advice but this well-dressed man had managed to convince them that he was a genuine expert. It was not too long before the seizures returned in full force . . . and the parents told their story.

In the past, promises of instant cures (using scare tactics), epilepsy remedies, nerve syrups, and nerve tonics were often sold by mail orders. Although this is less common nowadays, it still exists. Megavitamin therapy, faith healing, manipulation of the spine, acupuncture, and old-home remedies unfortunately cannot replace antiepileptic medications. Genuine, natural foods and low sugar diets have become popular and for very good reasons. As discussed above earlier, however, only the ketogenic diet is occasionally used by physicians in treating children with certain types of intractable epilepsy.

Sometimes there are no easy answers for stopping difficult seizures. In such situations and when suggestions for cures are received, parents should openly discuss them with the physician they have learned to trust.

Protective Helmets

When children have drop seizures, the loss of posture is so rapid that they may fall violently and crash to the ground. Because this type of epilepsy is often difficult to control by medications, the afflicted individuals are constantly exposed to physical injury. The unsightly facial scars, broken teeth, thickened lips, and swollen and bruised cheeks can be prevented through the wearing of a simple, specially adapted hockey helmet. If the child's head is too large, too small, or different in shape, most hospital occupational therapists or brace shops can adjust it, placing padding inside and adding pieces for chin and facial protection (Figure 1). Parents often decorate the helmets of younger children with pictures of flowers, animals, or cartoons. This way they are psychologically easier to wear.

What to Do for Accidental Overdosage

Valerie, who was 3 years old, day after day enviously watched her older brother swallow beautifully colored pills. One morning, only seconds after her mother had selected and carefully counted out the required number of tablets, she snatched them and before her mother could stop her, swallowed them all. This lead to frantic telephone calls, a frightened mother and a very sleepy Valerie.

It is of great importance for parents to know the possible side effects of antiepileptic medications and the symptoms of overdosage. When the child with epilepsy (or a sibling) takes one or two extra pills, there is little danger although the parents should discuss this with their physician as soon as possible.

In case of a marked overdosage, when the child is still alert he or she should be made to swallow undiluted evaporated milk, or as a second choice, ordinary milk. A spoonful of Ipecac syrup, which causes vomiting after a few minutes, should be given. Alternatively, vomiting may be induced by pushing a finger far back into the throat; with younger children this procedure may carry the danger of a bite. The next step is to give Activated Charcoal. (Syrup of Ipecac and Activated Charcoal with instructions should be kept in every household with small children.)

During the initial time period after overdose ingestion, every second counts. Parents must immediately call their physician who most likely will direct them to the nearest emergency ward for tests and observation. In case the physician is not available the parents should call the nearest hospital; most major hospitals have Poison

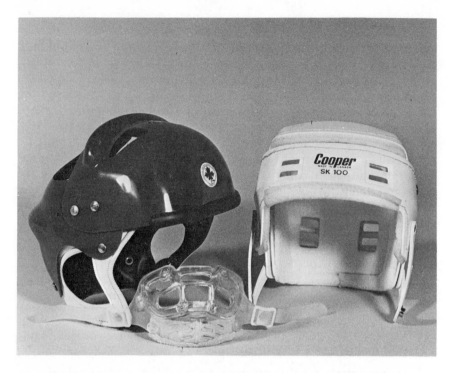

Figure 1.   Helmets are occasionally needed for children with uncontrolled epilepsy to protect their head and face from sudden falls.

Control Centers, offering immediate information and advice. The remaining medicine and the empty bottles should be brought in for identification.

When a child is unconscious, it is a dire emergency. An ambulance must be called immediately and nothing should be given by mouth because, due to impaired swallowing, it could be aspirated into the lungs. In the hospital, by inserting a tube through the nose into the stomach the contents are washed out. Life supportive systems, special intravenous medications, and the expert help of professional teams may also be used.

How to Give Medications to an Uncooperative Child

Sometimes small or retarded children refuse to take their medications. Mainly for psychological reasons they object to swallowing tablets or capsules. Pills can be crushed and mixed in with jam or honey. Many anticonvulsants are also available in liquid forms but in rare cases, children refuse liquid preparations as well, even though the unpleasant taste is disguised with strawberry or cherry flavors. This situation may result in a power struggle, which must be won by the parents. The parents must be careful, however, when uncooperative children are being forced to swallow something as they may choke on it.

Fortunately, parents eventually find ways to convince their children. If they do not, they must learn to safely administer medications in much the same way as medical students are taught to examine the throat or ears of a struggling child. The parent sits with the child on her lap. With her arms she tightly holds him, then with one hand she presses between his jaws so that the mouth opens up and with the other hand she squirts in the medicine (syringe is the best). Not a drop is spilled! When a child is sitting, rather than lying down, there is no danger of aspiration. If parents are still unable to manage, they can ask hospital nurses on pediatric wards, who are expert at this. These nurses will often point out that the main reason why most children refuse to take their medications is because of the hesitant and apprehensive attitude of the parents.

Some children just do not like taking their pills no matter what— perhaps for psychological reasons or because they are very sensitive to their taste.

Others transfer their anger about being sick onto the medicine. In either case parents need to be firm and clear: "I know you don't like this stuff but you have to take it!" Rewards or punishments should usually not be used. Like getting up and getting dressed, taking medication is a fact of life.

If a major struggle develops, it may signal a deeper problem that should be discussed with someone who has studied child and family development and child psychology. When parents have a clue why their children have a bad feeling about the medicine, they should bring it up during another time of the day when they are both comfortable. For instance, sounding them out with a questioning statement like, "it's tough to have an extra job like taking medicine every day" can provide a way for the children to begin to express their particular feelings. For younger children a parent's calm and firm approach will suffice. Even if they do not seem to react to or resist taking medications, asking about their feelings is important in maintaining communication and understanding. This will prepare them to be better patients later.

chapter 9

What to Do during a Convulsion

How Parents Are Introduced to Epilepsy

Basic Rules

Important Observations during a Seizure

Should the Ambulance Be Called?

Should the Doctor Be Phoned?

How Can Long Seizures Be Stopped when
 Doctors and Hospitals Are Too Far Away?

How Parents Are Introduced to Epilepsy

Most seizures last only for a few seconds or minutes although, to the parents, they seem like hours. As discussed above, the pattern of epilepsy varies markedly from person to person. There are convulsive and non-convulsive seizures.

There is nothing more terrifying for parents than to witness their child's first convulsion. Few have seen a seizure before and most have misconceived notions about epilepsy.

George Tibor was 4 years old when he had his first seizure. The day before his attack he had not been feeling well—had had a dry cough, fever and a poor appetite. Late next morning his mother heard gurgling noises in the living room, ran in and found George on the floor. He was stiff, ash-colored and unconscious. He did not seem to be breathing so at first she thought he had choked on something. She tried prying open his tightly closed jaws and in this attempt had her finger bitten; she then tried to push a spoon between his teeth but that did not work—in fact, she chipped one of his teeth. Frantically, she ran next door for help. The neighbor called an ambulance and took over the care of Mrs. Tibor's other child.

Five or six minutes later when the ambulance arrived, George was breathing more regularly but he was in a deep sleep. It was in the emergency ward that the attending physician told Mrs. Tibor that George had had a seizure and probably had epilepsy.

Basic Rules

A simple staring spell like in petit mal epilepsy may be so short that there is no time for intervention. When the spell is longer, for instance, in complex partial seizures, the children may be out of touch with reality although still partially aware. In these cases the parents should try to make them comfortable but must not restrain them as they may resist violently. They should be observed carefully but with minimal interference unless an accident is likely to occur. Talking and asking questions is a useful way to check on the level of their consciousness. They should not be forced to swallow an extra tablet or capsule because anticonvulsants, due to their delayed action, do not immediately become effective. Furthermore, choking on the medicine is a real danger.

Convulsions can be terrifying but the parents must try to keep calm. Children are best placed on a bed, or a couch, or left on the floor where they cannot hurt themselves. The body should be turned on the side and the head supported in a way that it is partially facing the floor. In this position the saliva that is often produced in excess during a convulsion will not obstruct the airways (Figure 1). It is not possible to swallow one's tongue, as many people incorrectly believe. Occasionally, during or after a seizure a child will vomit; lying on one side will prevent the choking and for the same reason, in this position, the saliva freely flows out of the child's mouth and will not accumulate in the back of the throat. The clothing should be loosened and if worn glasses, these should be removed.

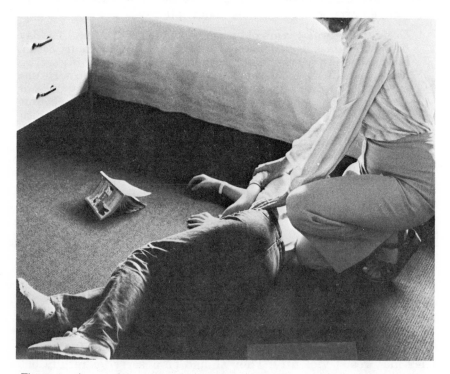

Figure 1.   A convulsing child should be placed on his or her side, protected from injury.

There is no need to place anything in the mouth unless in exceptionally rare cases when it is specified by the physician (Figure 2). The hard objects may injure the teeth and soft ones inevitably reduce the airway. If there is tongue biting, this likely happens at the very onset of a convulsion—with the first clenching of the jaw. Often people who are coming to the aid of a convulsing person feel that the only way they can help is to stop the jerking. They may even sit on the moving body but restraining not only doesn't help but may cause injury. It is a good idea to protect the head by holding it or having it rest on a pillow or on some clothing if the attack occurs in the street.

When the temperature of a young child is elevated and the convulsion is presumably febrile in nature, the body needs to be sponged off and kept cool as described earlier.

After the convulsion, due to the "exhaustion" that follows such a storm of the nervous system, the child goes into a deep sleep. This

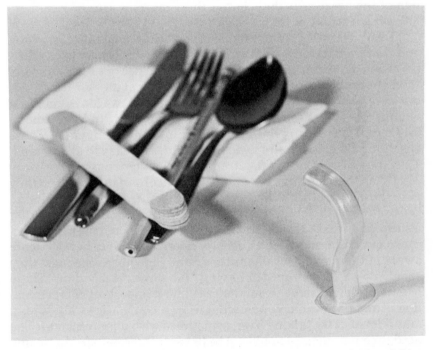

Figure 2.   Objects should not be placed between the teeth of a convulsing child.

should no longer be considered part of the seizure but rather a natural consequence of it—the so called "post-ictal" period. If the child has fallen to the ground during the convulsion, many "inexperienced" parents fear that drowsiness and post-ictal sleep is due to a concussion. This occurs only with a very severe head injury. The child should be allowed to sleep and usually, gradually wakes up in 15 to 30 minutes. There is no need to stimulate the child with coffee, tea, or water as it would still be easy to choke on liquids.

After a convulsion, most children are tired, cranky, and lethargic, often for the remainder of the day. They may even have splitting headaches (for which pain relievers can be given) and have no recollections of previous events. On occasion after awakening, one side of the body, an arm or a leg (usually where the convulsion was the strongest) can be weak for a few minutes or up to several hours. This important observation should be reported to the doctor. It is known as *Todd's paralysis* and is not caused by a stroke but by the exhaustion of the nerve cells that control these muscles. Unlike weakness following a stroke, it is transient.

Every seizure may remind everyone that something is wrong and that there is a continuing medical problem. It may evoke fear, heightened awareness, a sense of wanting to flee or to dramatically solve the problem (to do something), and anger at the "attack." Once the convulsion is over, guilty worries ("Did we do something wrong?") or even a sense of anger toward the child ("Why did she do this to us?") or ("Why did he do it again?") may linger on. These questions are emotionally logical, natural, and easy to understand. They may also occur in other troublesome situations.

Often these feelings get confusing or are hard to face. Then they may show up in other ways, such as, exaggerated irritation or indulgence toward the child, marital or parenting conflicts over other issues. That these emotions can be so intense is not surprising because our children affect us deeply. Even as parents become more aware of their own as well as other family members' feelings, they should not be discouraged at having "the same old reaction." These reactions should serve as reminders of how important communication is and of how much we need it after a traumatic event. It may take a lot of extra talking over, sometimes with a professional. The need to communicate should not be turned off. To be "strong" is fine but part of being truly strong is being able to recognize, bear, and share our own emotions.

Important Observations during a Seizure

Each time the child is in the doctor's office, the physician will be asking the family for a detailed description of the seizures. Parents can help by giving accurate information. Therefore, they should make objective observations and keep records of the episodes, although not in an overzealous, excessive manner. Such a "seizure calendar" could be a regular calendar or a simple note book. Each page is used to record a particular month in a year. At the top of the page is the month, the year, and the name and amounts of the medications. Then three columns are made—in the first is the specific date, in the second column the type and duration of seizures, and in the third, any possible associations. The following observations are helpful:

The number and duration of seizures since the last visit, the day and hour they occurred.
What was the child doing at the time?
Was the child drowsy, overtired, or had he or she missed medications?
Was there a warning sign (aura)? How did it progress?
Did he or she cry out?
Where did the twitching start, was it the same on both sides?
Did the eyes turn, roll, or twitch? Did the head turn? Which way?
Was the child stiff, limp, or have an unusual posture?
Did he or she blink rhythmically or swallow during the seizure?
Was behavior automatic or repetitive?
Was the child conscious, unconscious, or confused?
Did speech change during or after? Did he or she say anything?
Was the child dizzy, nauseated, and did he or she vomit? Did the child complain of a headache?
Was the child's face pale, red, or blue at the onset, during or after the attack?
Was the child incontinent?
Did the child go to sleep after the seizure?

No one can remember all the details but it is surprising how much parents can recall when they are questioned specifically.

It is important for parents to understand what consciousness is. It is an awareness of one's surroundings and an ability to respond. Children who have retained their consciousness during a seizure subsequently can tell what has happened and what questions were asked. Unconsciousness is not the same as the loss of posture or the inability to stand up. Therefore, after falling to the ground children may remain fully aware. When speech is lost during the attack there are those who are able to respond by gestures rather than verbally. Some are mute while others merely have automatic speech and answer questions in repetitive sentences: "Do you feel well?" "I am ok, I am ok." Children may mumble words totally out of context without any recollection afterward. Some may remember the events immediately before and after but not during the seizure.

Should the Ambulance Be Called?

During the first few seizures, parents inevitably tend to call the ambulance or the police and their child is rushed to the hospital. Later, when they become less panicky and more familiar with the patterns of epilepsy these calls seem to become not so necessary.

The seizures represent traumatic experiences for the family. To the children they are more traumatic if they wake up in an ambulance or a hospital, not knowing what has happened. However, when the attacks are strong, last longer than 20 to 30 minutes, or when one convulsion follows another, it is mandatory to bring the child, even by family car, to the nearest emergency ward. There, life supporting systems and particularly intravenous medications to control the seizures are available. In addition a child with epilepsy may have sustained a cut that needs to be sutured. Obviously, the severity of seizures, the location of the family, the health and age of the child, and many other factors influence the decision as to whether they should be taken to hospitals. Parents should always discuss with their physician what they should do in case of a convulsion and they should be prepared for emergencies.

Should the Doctor Be Phoned?

Parents must use common sense in judging when it is appropriate to call their doctors. They also have to understand the difference between the family physician and the specialist who was consulted. Some doctors, like the pediatrician may wish to be notified each time the child has a seizure. All doctors will feel upset when they are called with insignificant complaints even if this is done during the day. Judgment and education are essential factors. A good relationship is based on mutual respect and trust with the understanding that doctors are busy and responsible for many medical problems and that the welfare of the child is the main concern of the parents. A thorough discussion with the physician is the key to parents knowing when they are free to call. "Insignificant" or "major" events depend upon one's point of view. It is only through gradual education and explanation that a parent can learn what the doctor believes to be "insignificant" or "major." To a parent, a small seizure may be significantly troublesome while apparent sleepiness for 2 days may not be major. To the physician, it may be just the opposite.

How Can Long Seizures Be Stopped when Doctors and Hospitals Are Too Far Away?

Occasionally a child with epilepsy lives far from medical facilities and in case of a prolonged seizure, the parents must be able to offer some treatment. In such situations parents can be taught to give intramuscular medications. It is not difficult to give a shot of Valium in the buttock or thigh although the technique must be carefully taught, and the dose supervised.

Rectally administered medications offer an even better alternative because they are rapidly absorbed into the blood stream. Intravenous Valium, which is stored in vials, can be used for rectal administration. The neck of the vial is broken (it is a good idea to use a tissue paper so the fingers are not cut) and the required amount drawn up into a small syringe. The needle is removed, the tip of the syringe is fitted with a small rubber or plastic tube which is then inserted 1″ to 1½″ into the rectal passage. Then the liquid medication is instilled from the syringe into the rectum (Figure 3). Similarly, paraldehyde can also be given rectally but because it is more irritating than Valium it should be mixed with two parts of olive oil or mineral oil. However, paraldehyde must be well preserved and freshly prepared a short time before by the local pharmacist. Occasionally, even crushed oral diazepam tablets, as prescribed by the doctor, can be given especially when there are frequently recurring seizures. In rare cases when a child is predisposed to long and severe seizures, the parents may be trained to administer oxygen from a tank that is kept at home.

When parents live far away from medical facilities they should plan what they will do in case of emergencies. Nothing is worse than helplessly watching a child convulse for several hours with the realization that long and severe seizures can be damaging. The treat-

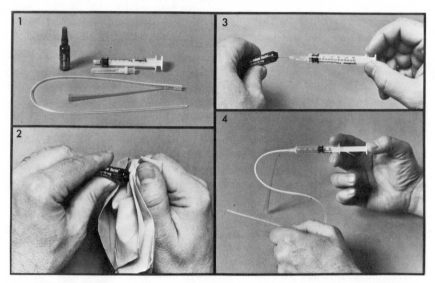

Figure 3.   This picture sequence shows how to administer rectal Valium.

ment that can be given by parents, the route of administration, dose, and frequency must be carefully discussed and rehearsed with the physician, clinic nurses, or hospital.

chapter 10

The Early Years

Childhood Illnesses
Immunization
Babysitting
Identifying Chains and Bracelets
Sleeping Arrangements
Swimming and Bathing
Traveling
Entering School

Childhood Illnesses

When children with epilepsy are sick, there is a greater chance for them to have seizures. In fact during a febrile illness the blood levels of some anticonvulsants may drop slightly. Unrelated to this, parents frequently wonder whether cough syrups, aspirin, antihistamines, antibiotics, or other medications can safely be given to a child who is on anticonvulsant treatment. Each newly added drug for the infection, cough, or fever to some extent can interfere with the absorption, circulation, and elimination of the other. Now that medications can be measured in the blood, doctors are just beginning to understand the extremely complex drug interactions. There are still many unanswered questions. For practical purposes when necessary parents can safely administer the usual remedies and this should be discussed with the physician.

Children who have just vomited their medication, should get another dose but when they have stomach disturbances and are unable to keep anything down, the parents must immediately notify the physician. If recurrent vomiting is not stopped by suppositories, these children may need to be admitted to a hospital where intravenous or intramuscular administration of the anticonvulsant will tide them over that period of illness.

Immunization

Immunizing a child who has seizures should be discussed with the physician. Epilepsy is not a contraindication unless steroids are used in the treatment. It is a common misconception that handicapped children may sustain brain damage if they are immunized against some of the childhood illnesses. This is not so. The consequences of whooping cough, measles, small pox, polio, or diphtheria are far worse than the occasional complication from immunization. The only concern is that the febrile reaction that often follows the shot may trigger a convulsion and precautions should be taken accordingly.

Babysitting

When, during a meeting, parents of handicapped children were requested to list their major problems, they mentioned babysitting as their number one concern. Teenage girls, who are most often asked to do this job, are reluctant and afraid. Yet the parents must make an effort to go out together for a social evening, to a movie, or just for a walk once or twice a week. Otherwise they become chronically tired and "burned out." It is when medical problems are intense that taking a break becomes most important.

Getting a babysitter for the parents whose child's epilepsy is not well-controlled is difficult. To witness and manage a convulsing person or one who becomes markedly irritable and hostile after a seizure is frightening and a big responsibility. It is not surprising, therefore, that even professional babysitting agencies often decline their services for children with epilepsy. Most families are fortunate in having relatives or friends who will help. If not, parents who belong to local epilepsy associations often babysit for one another; at other times volunteers attached to these organizations are available. After securing the services of a babysitter the parents must openly discuss their child's epilepsy. They should leave clear instructions on what to do in the event of a seizure and where they or their physician can be reached.

Identifying Chains and Bracelets

The purpose of chains and bracelets that identify a person as having epilepsy is to assist helpers in recognizing the medical problem and in quickly initiating appropriate management. Such identification may be redundant for younger children as they are rarely without the supervision of their parents, relatives, teachers, babysitters, or others who already know their medical condition. Furthermore, the treatment which would be beneficial to physicians coming in contact with them during emergencies, is not mentioned. Identifying devices are more useful for independent adolescents, who could carry a card stating they have epilepsy, listing the medications and their doses. Such information provided to bystanders, police officers at the site of the emergency, or to hospital staff can avoid unnecessary investigations, unfortunate mishaps, or misunderstandings. Drug abuse, alcoholism, and criminal offenses are often suspected. In some states, however, officers are not allowed to look in wallets. Chains and bracelets can be obtained from most pharmacies (Medic Alert) and the physician can supply a card with the appropriate information.

Sleeping Arrangements

Sometimes seizures occur at night and during daytime naps, often soon after falling asleep or upon awakening. Understandably, children with epilepsy should not sleep in a top bunk bed because they may fall out during a convulsion. Their rooms should be near to their parents but sleeping in the parents' bedrooms, or beds, must be discouraged. Young children with generalized convulsions probably should have a firm mattress and a hard pillow to prevent the remote possibility of smothering during their seizure and the deep sleep that follows. It is just not possible and not realistic to watch over children every second, day and night. Too much anxiety creates excessive dependence and the fact that an attack during sleep may be missed has to be accepted. Fortunately nocturnal seizures generally do not last long. If the seizure is severe and the child is sleeping in a room next to the parents, it will not be missed. Parents may feel more secure using wireless, sensitive plug-in intercoms so they can hear their child's activities even during the night. The intercoms are relatively cheap, portable, and can be used with any electrical outlet.

Swimming and Bathing

It is common sense that children with certain types of epilepsy should not be allowed to swim without strict supervision. The most appropriate site for them to swim is a pool under the watchful eye of life guards or responsible adults. The attendants should be prepared to help in case of a seizure. Under these circumstances there is no danger and no need for restrictions. Drowning can also occur in bathtubs so certain rules must be observed; these apply mainly to older children because infants are supervised anyway. Bathing when alone in the house should be avoided. When a youngster takes a bath the door should not be locked. It is safer to use as little water as possible so that the face will remain above water level if he or she is lying down. But all these precautions will not prevent a catastrophe if the child falls unconscious face down without making a sound to attract attention. For this reason taking a shower is safer than a bath although injuries can still occur. To avoid bad burns the temperature of the water should be just comfortably warm, not hot, and a person with frequent seizures could sit on a stool while taking a shower. Fortunately in many cases of epilepsy these precautions are not necessary; anticipating this sort of problem depends on the parents' knowledge regarding their child's epilepsy.

Traveling

Parents are often anxious about taking their child with epilepsy on long trips. When the seizures are reasonably well-controlled, traveling by car or airplane is safe although excessive tiredness should be avoided. An adequate supply of medication must be brought and if the attacks are the grand mal type or prolonged, parents should be prepared for emergencies. It is worthwhile to have copies of the medical records as these can be very helpful in emergencies. Rectal Valium or paraldehyde may also be carried and used (see Chapter 9). Long trips should be discussed with the physician who may give special recommendations, an extra prescription or a medical statement.

Entering School

When a child with epilepsy goes to school, the parents are wise to discuss the medical aspects with the teachers and the principal. The school nurse will also have to be informed about the type, frequency, and severity of the seizures and the medication. Witnessing a convulsion is upsetting to those who have never seen it before. Therefore, not only the teachers but also the students in the class need to be prepared if that child is likely to have a seizure. The teachers cannot be expected to be knowledgeable on all handicaps, therefore, the parents and the nurse must educate them further with pamphlets or books on epilepsy. The local epilepsy societies should have a list of suitable material. Comic books and films are also available for students.

One of the major problems students with epilepsy encounter is the lack of acceptance by their peers. Many complain that they are shunned by their classmates who may be frightened by unexpected, sudden "involuntary behavior," a seizure. In the past, schools were so apprehensive about having students with epilepsy that their enrollment was often refused. This is no longer so. School personnel can be extremely helpful although education of children with frequent seizures is still a hardship for all concerned.

> The Logans did not wish to inform the school about the seizure disorder of their son, Donald. They felt that confidential records often leak out and that this might prejudice Donald's future. Besides, a child's health is not a teacher's concern. Two months later Donald unexpectedly had a convulsion in class, and everyone was horrified. An ambulance was called and Donald woke up in the emergency ward of the nearest hospital. The teachers and the principal were very resentful because the parents had withheld important information about Donald's health. Mr. and Mrs. Logan regretfully learned their lesson. After all, a child's health is the teacher's concern too!

Until a few years ago, antiepileptic medications were administered at regular intervals three or four times a day; the parents had to send the noon medication to the school to be administered by the teacher or the school nurse. This should, whenever possible, be avoided. It is understandable that teachers may dislike giving medications; it creates an additional concern and they may feel that this is not their job. In many states there are legal restrictions and the school periodically has to be notified in writing by the doctor. It is now well-proven that anticonvulsants do not need to be given at absolutely exact intervals; in most cases if the doses are tolerated they can simply be taken in the morning and at night. When children still have to take their medicine three times a day, one dose can be given right after they return from school.

Some anticonvulsants tend to dull awareness and motivation and cause excessive tiredness. Usually, adjusting the dose with the guidance of the blood levels alleviates this problem. Occasionally, physicians may use a stimulant, such as Ritalin to counteract the sedative side-effects. In general, however, everyone would agree that it is better for a child to take less medication (although there is a chance of an occasional seizure) than to be so oversedated that learning is severely impaired. Fortunately, there are now more anticonvulsants available that cause little or no sedation. This is an important consideration in selecting drugs. When the parents or teachers feel that the treatment adversely affects the child's school performance, this should be brought to the attention of the physician.

The teacher's expectations of children with epilepsy must be realistic. One teacher fought against the enrollment of a student who had seizures and then completely ignored the child. His expectation of that child was nil. He believed that persons with epilepsy were brain damaged and that they were not capable of learning. He felt that such students should be in a special class with the mentally retarded. This type of attitude must be corrected. It is true, however, that many children with seizures have learning problems (see Chapter 13).

> Tom's grade 4 teacher thought that even the slightest stress might bring on a seizure and, therefore, she avoided asking him questions, gave no assignments and handled him very gingerly. As a result, Tom was having a wonderful time but he was just not learning much. His mother, who had already raised two children, sensed that something was wrong in school and had a good talk with the teacher—correcting her attitude.

Although it is true that excessive stress may be a factor in triggering some seizures, this does not apply to the type of pressure most children with epilepsy may experience in school. The teacher's reaction to epilepsy not only influences the child's own self-perception but also the attitude of his or her peers. Many teachers are hesitant in talking to parents about the child's seizures and especially about their own feeling. They should be encouraged to do so by the parents themselves.

Children with epilepsy should not be totally excluded from physical education. Healthy activity, as compared to idleness, reduces the chance for seizures and participation helps to develop their self-confidence. Students with frequent epileptic attacks should not participate in certain activities such as rope climbing and use of high bars, but running, baseball, and many other sports need to be encouraged (see Chapter 12). If necessary, the parents could give the school a witnessed letter of consent absolving the teachers from any blame when during physical education due to a seizure a student sustains an injury. The education of teachers about epilepsy is obviously most important.

chapter 11

The Impact of Epilepsy: Common Feelings and Complications

The Child
Common Feelings
The Parents
The Siblings
The Family Network

The writing of this book has been stimulated by the authors' belief that the first rule in the treatment of epilepsy is the creation of a partnership with the parents—a partnership requiring mutual respect. Physicians show this through their sharing information and their clinical wisdom. Seizures teach us that no one answer is final in facing the unpredictable. This book provides a separate opportunity —away from the tensions of office and hospital visits—for understanding epilepsy. Questions can be focused, asked again, and refined, and answers can be digested slowly. The knowledge gained will help parents provide the best care for the children and will also help the parents coordinate the efforts of other helpers.

Throughout these chapters, clinical information and common reactions to the diagnosis of epilepsy are emphasized. The description of feelings is provided to allow family members to recognize and accept them. Trying to ignore or deny these natural feelings (which occur when a child develops epilepsy) can make things worse, as can giving in to fears and uncertainties. It can be difficult to hold to a middle ground. There are times when we need to endure our thoughts while at other times they can prompt us to seek changes.

All solutions have their good and bad sides but they are rarely, if ever, perfect. For example, a child may cry when the parents leave. If the problem is solved by the parents always staying home, the positive result is that the youngster does not cry. The negative aspect may be the creation of a belief in the child's mind that it is impossible to be left alone. Both short-term and long-term effects need to be considered. It is difficult to make decisions without discussions and questions.

Unlike a minor injury, epilepsy has many uncertainties. The cause is often obscure. The treatment needs to be tailored to each individual—it may change periodically or it may last for years. Therefore, the medical guideline, "the best possible control with least side effects," must be balanced with the human objective of accepting difficulties while fostering both the strength and independence of the child. During this process, common feelings and reactions can be experienced by all concerned.

The Child

When Chris, a 10-year-old with epilepsy, heard that this book was being written, he asked to be included. He explained that his story was important. He wanted other kids to know that he had to learn how to deal with his seizures and also that he had discovered that a talking doctor could help him do it. Chris thought most kids find it hard to admit they have epilepsy, even to themselves, and that they are bothered by their feelings about it. He was glad to hear that his thoughts are common and he hoped other kids would realize this too.

Chris was sad, mad, and scared. He was sad and mad because he didn't like and didn't want his seizures. Sometimes he was angry because he couldn't give his spells to someone else, like Bill—his "favorite enemy." Then even thinking this way became frustrating as Chris felt guilty about having these thoughts. Although he had only had a few seizures in his life he was scared because his epilepsy might come at the least expected time; nevertheless, he didn't like to admit his fears. He was somewhat of a perfectionist and this didn't help either—epilepsy was one more thing that certainly wasn't perfect!

To Chris, his mom and dad were very special so he didn't want them to feel badly about his epilepsy. He knew that they too were sometimes sad and scared and he worried that if he talked about his thoughts too much his parents would feel worse. It was a big relief to meet someone outside the family who could understand him and both reassure and help him talk more to his parents.

At the time when Chris first sat down to talk about the seizures his own feelings were more troublesome than the epilepsy itself. He felt worse following a convulsion at a movie in school. Because he was afraid of having further attacks he stopped going to the movies and, in general, was less willing to go out. He had trouble sleeping. He felt uncomfortable with his friends and was mad that no one in his family could "make it better." At the age of 10, Chris was dealing with a new sense of awareness about his epilepsy and his feelings about it.

At each developmental stage, the effects of having epilepsy vary. For the preschooler this means disliking the taste of the medicine, a reaction to an unfamiliar medical setting or being frustrated because of the need to lie still for the EEG. The information parents give acts as a buffer for these experiences and begins to build a foundation for later awareness. When preschoolers are sad, mad, or scared, they will show it. It is only when these feelings are not clearly acknowledged and comfort not offered that complications can occur.

One of the more troublesome complications in the life of preschoolers often develops from the parents' reactions to the seizures. When the anxiety and distress of the parents begin to affect how limits are set or how separation is tolerated, these children may start having behavioral problems and/or difficulties with anxiety. All parents are scared and distressed when epilepsy is diagnosed; however, they cannot let these feelings "make things worse." They must allow their children to develop a sense of independence and learn the basic rules of behavior.

Once the routines of tests, doctor's visits, EEGs, medications, and the rest are mastered, children (unless there are other problems such as developmental delays, hyperactivity, attentional or learning difficulties) usually do as well in accepting their epilepsy as their parents. Sometimes they manage even better. In middle childhood and early adolescence, however, children become aware of their medical problems in new ways. They may get angry when they see that epilepsy does not go away and scared when they realize the implications of taking medicine away from home. They feel sad again about "being stuck" unfairly with their seizure disorder. Now a new level of acceptance and knowledge must be fashioned. Sometimes when parents see their children wrestling with these problems they are tempted to suppress their thoughts ("Let's not talk about it. Think of cheerful things.") because they may believe that if you can't change it, ignore it. Children often need to sort through their feelings about epilepsy before they can ignore them again.

In addition to dealing with the consequences of seizures, children between 8 and 13 years of age also need to deal realistically with other associated handicaps. They must also learn that no matter how much they wish, mom, dad, and the doctors cannot make them go away. The parents, like the medical team, need to be able to "tell it like it is" no matter how hard this is. The following story illustrates this.

> Al, an 11-year-old, is the older of two boys from an Italian-American family. He had a mixed seizure disorder since his preschool years. Along with his troublesome epileptic attacks he experienced problems with coordination and learning arithmetic. He felt badly about his difficulties and was aware of the pressure to achieve in his family system. Individual and family treatment was started in order to help him deal with the sense of incompetence that had begun to develop. Model making served as a focus for the treatment sessions; working on a project would challenge his patience, expose his difficulty in following instructions, and highlight some of the troubles with coordination.
>
> Al loved cars and making auto models. However, model building at home had been a source of frustration for him since his younger brother did it with so much more ease. While working together was stressful it provided an opportunity for the psychiatrist to review the above issues and show Al how, in many instances, his feelings and reactions caused further difficulties.

In the course of the model building it became clear again how sensitive an issue competence is. It took a couple of sessions to work on the engine and then to mount it on the chassis. At one point Al declared, "Let's leave these out," referring to two plastic supports that went somewhere alongside the engine. Since he was in charge (and as it was, enough struggles had occurred on that day), his request was granted. Later in the month he finished assembling the body of the car and was ready to put the two pieces together. After he left that day one could see that the fit was very poor. During the next 2 or 3 days the psychiatrist kept continually wishing that he could quietly sneak back and patch things up so that it would be "easier" for Al and the model would "look better." There he was debating a behind-the-scenes patch-up job, knowing how many hours he had spent unravelling the complications that resulted from this family's unrealistic expectations. On the one hand they distorted the feedback that they gave their epileptic son and on the other hand they had asked him to do the impossible.

The point of this anecdote is to remind us what a powerful stimulus chronic medical problems can exert on the family and on other involved caregivers. Distortions of feedback affect the development of children's sense of autonomy (the ability to exert influence in the personal and interpersonal environment) and their sense of competence (the ability to have command over the inanimate world). These distortions in feedback occur again and again.

During the later teenage years, similar thoughts (it's unfair, can't be fixed?) and associated feelings (anger, dismay, and others) are experienced. Depending upon the degree of seizure control or the severity of other handicaps, the questions related to a driver's license and the acceptance of others (dating) become prominent concerns. These reflect the adolescent's desire for independence, self-respect and wishes for the future. As painful as it may be, these thoughts and feelings need to be heard within the family circle and discussed. Often it is particularly helpful to air these issues with a counselor because each person in a family may have different feelings as well as different styles of coping.

Chris, like other youngsters, had to face his worries and feelings and figure out a new way of coping. As he said, "I had to learn that I was mad, sad, and scared. And no matter how much I wanted to, I couldn't give it to Bill! I was glad I could talk it over with someone."

Common Feelings

Just as children experience a set of feelings in response to their epilepsy, the other members of the family also have expected reactions. These include sadness, a sense of helplessness, anger, and guilt.

Sadness affects everyone in the family and it never quite goes away. It is not always fully present but unexpected seizures, difficulties at school or the reaction of a friend may bring it back.

The *helplessness* that each member of the family may experience is slightly different. No one can make the epileptic disorder go away or can prevent additional pressures. All of them may feel distressed about the change brought on by the seizures as things will not return to normal. When there is less support available people are more helpless about managing the burden and its emotional complications. Everyone in the family can help each other cope. This difficulty is certainly heightened in single parent families.

Anger is commonly felt. One child said, "I've been angry ever since I was a little kid; I always felt I shouldn't be and that I should be good. After all, my brother was sick and nobody else was mad." These children often feel unbearably alone with this anger. What makes siblings so angry? Unfortunately it is the same thing that has made everyone else depressed, withdrawn, critical of doctors, hopeful, or denying the problem. One source of anger is from their sense of deprivation. They lose out on things they want and feel chronically neglected. "I didn't always want to be quiet or good but there was nothing else I could do to change Bill's coming first. I'd always be second. There was no way to compete with Bill's sickness." One upset father said this about his son even though he knew his wife couldn't have managed things better. Mothers feel angry that others don't help out more. No wonder it can be so hard to discuss what to do.

The siblings' anger is associated with their belief that there is less parental caregiving and attention and the perception of all the extra goodies the ill child gets. This may make it harder for them to ask for what they want or make them less willing to help out. They feel angry about everyone keeping quiet about what they need because of the seizures. "Whenever I've had to ask for something I really wanted, I'd get frightened (of the underlying anger). When I was little, I just decided I would never tell anyone what I wanted when I was really angry." The withholding of 'self' is then experienced as a proper punishment for the "neglectful" others.

Guilt follows anger. It is natural to feel guilty when everybody is so angry. One mother said, "I was afraid of hearing myself saying those angry things deep in my heart. I was disappointed in everyone." It is difficult to have such deep resentment in the presence of genuine love and not feel guilty about it. This often results in further defense mechanisms such as efforts to be good, not asking for help, and self denial. One sister stated, "I tried not to give my parents more pain than they already had but it was hard to keep being so good."

This guilt can be compared to the feelings of survivors who remain alive after a disaster while others died. Others in the family are well, one is not. Guilt may also relate to the wish these individuals have to take care of themselves just as the survivors related their guilt to actions they had taken to save themselves. Other family members tried to survive. They are not sick and everyone still tries to have a good time.

Guilt may also be associated with all the normal pleasures of life, like going out, dancing, having friends, and enjoying things. One healthy sibling remarked about his handicapped brother, "There he was, in bed. He couldn't walk; it was hard for him to eat. I felt there were other things I wanted to do besides sitting there and feeling guilty."

The Parents

The birth of most children is an affirmation of hope, human caregiving, and love. It is a connection to both past and future. Newborns are the blossoming of wishes, which can represent an answer for past losses and regrets. Now, in the future they may stimulate barely conscious fantasies about oneself or turn previous despairs into realistic and unrealistic hopes.

At the same time there is danger. The child's presence may wrap up all the fears and the rarely admitted unkind thoughts. These may first strike a parent during the infant's normal crying spells or rages. They can instantaneously percolate down into the secret well of one's own torments. Parents survive these moments. Everyone longs for them to be distant and short lived but on occasion, they are not. Illness, developmental delay, or injury can tax the fragile alliance we have with our humaneness. That feeling is particularly intense when the newborn child is delivered with a built-in "mistake" (a birth defect). It is a starkly defined reminder of our own basic biology.

The independent North American parents live in a community that they ordinarily fence off by filling their houses with things so there will be no need to borrow. These "independent" parents may look into the crib of a convulsing or deformed child with loneliness and a new longing for a place in the human community. They are reminded to recreate a community of sharing.

Questions have always been asked and we have answered them one way or another. Although scientific data greatly proliferated, the reasons of the heart vary little. Most pertinent to the burden that the parent of a handicapped child will carry is this life-long *why*. Through the centuries the parents were always blamed. . . . The problem was their fault. It is not surprising, therefore, that these children from the onset of their epilepsy make their mothers and fathers feel guilty. Their cries make parents think of their own deficiencies and failures. Then sorrow and rage can follow.

What allows parents to survive? It is the network of support that is found in families and friends. The distance between mothers and fathers and their place of work, the separation between one's home and the community, the gap between the nuclear family and the extended, are all hard to bridge. Society does not now support the growth of the family fabric within the community. Economic policy does not yet foster the development of a workplace that promotes the well being of the entire family. It is a job still to be done.

A chronic disorder of a child can disrupt family life in different ways. On a basic day-to-day level, the physical set-up of the household, meal-planning, and the distribution of parental time, are all affected. The more severe the problem, the greater are the stresses on the parents and, therefore, also on all other members. This in turn increases the emotional burden from the strain of anger and guilt. How parents manage these feelings can have a dramatic effect on the family. Communications may be shut down. Parents may withdraw emotionally in order to defend themselves from painful feelings. At stressful times irritation and disappointment are more easily expressed than other emotions.

The presence of uncontrolled epilepsy can exaggerate or exacerbate any pre-existing marital quarrels. Parents may become too attached to that child. This "skewed" relationship can contribute to their poor perception of the siblings' needs, or create a distorted view of each other's attitudes. The chronic stress on the marital unit can spark old frictions and alliances between parents and grandparents. This then may affect the grandparents' behavior with the children.

These are the dangers. They deserve to be emphasized so that parents can avoid these complications or can identify them in order to get help. In most families the child's medical problem provides an opportunity to increase communication and empathy. It also contributes to stronger ties with the family network and the community and it promotes the kind of intimacy that allows people to endure the difficulties.

The Siblings

The siblings of a child with epilepsy are in a precarious and difficult position. They are not the direct victims of that disorder but often helpless and deprived bystanders. The question Why has this happened to me? immediately comes to the mind of the afflicted child and parents. Although this is also a natural thought for the siblings, their right to question is often denied. The parents may say, "What do you mean, why has this happened to you? It *hasn't* happened to *you!* You should thank your lucky stars." But something has indeed happened to the siblings, and it needs to be recognized by both parents and counselors. They are victims of family circumstances, which moves them to the periphery of their parents' concern. Consequently, they have difficulty adapting.

The feelings of siblings and the nature of their support from the parents may be adversely affected by the fluctuating course of the medical disorder. The seizures do not take into account the extracurricular activities or school life of a brother or sister. The parents may not be able to tolerate their own helplessness, guilt, or anger, and may become extraordinarily sensitive to many displayed feelings on the part of the sibling. Normal interactions between children that involve jealousy, a desire for parental attention, competitiveness, and so forth, can all become distorted by the parents' projecttions so that the sibling is in a chronically disadvantaged position.

Unlike the afflicted child, who may find a challenge in dealing with the medical problems, the siblings are often alienated and frightened by their own feelings and the complex process that surrounds them. The child with epilepsy is encouraged to do things, and parents offer enriched experiences to that child. The siblings are told to understand when they can not participate. When their ability to be generous is already overtaxed, they are requested to accept the special privileges given to their brother or sister, often with no return. They are asked to join the "ill" child, when they wish and need to keep separate. These attitudes may exert a pervasive effect on their lives.

How does a brother or sister deal with this situation? Denial is one of the most familiar mechanisms. The siblings do not have epilepsy, they are adjacent to it. The afflicted child may be able to ward off or deny the impact of the seizures, but the siblings can be in the lonesome position of seeing it all too clearly. The coping mechanisms of the child with epilepsy can include intellectualization, identification with the medical staff, and idiosyncratic rituals that are used to master either the nature of the disorder or the treatment itself. These mechanisms are not as available for the siblings but can be fostered. Often they are excluded from discussions of the seizure disorder and treatment; therefore, their understanding is incomplete. This lack of adequate information increases their mystification and fear. Without help from skillful medical staff, their ability to find allies and objects of identification is decreased. Their wish for this aid is reflected by the observation that a number of siblings later select the "helping professions"—social work—as their career. Finally, the afflicted child's medical problems and emotional defenses blur into a mysterious process that is difficult for the siblings to understand, much less master.

On occasions, medical visits can be made into family trips. Then, everyone can see and hear what seizures are all about and how they are treated. New audio visual aids that families can watch together are being developed. Everyone should have a chance to find out what there is to know and to share how they feel so that all members of the family can work together as best they can.

The Family Network

A chronic medical disorder of a child may cause a subtle disconnection between the nuclear family, relatives, and neighbors. The family sees itself as awkward, guilty, an alien, intrusive outsider, or as a burden. Gradually people drift away and yet the family needs them to talk about their experiences. Unfortunately, discussing the problems and discontents created by the child's chronic handicap is often prohibited within and outside the family. Adults and youngsters alike are isolated with their experiences. To remark on "the abnormal" becomes too sensitive and too painful an issue and, finally, silently prohibited.

It takes work and time to keep channels of communication open within and outside the family, but it is a worthwhile investment. It allows everyone to gain something in dealing with a difficult situation.

chapter 12

Adolescence and Young Adulthood

Recreation, Sports, and Camping

Driving

Parties, Alcohol, Pot, and Smoking

Dating and Marriage

Pregnancy

Breastfeeding

Is Epilepsy Hereditary? Genetic Counseling

Insurance

Lay Epilepsy Organizations

The Rights of Children with Epilepsy in
 Education, Employment, and Health

Communication with Helpers

Suggested Reading

Recreation, Sports, and Camping

Healthy activity, as compared to idleness, reduces the chance of seizures. Although there are a few parents and grandparents who go to extremes in protecting a child's head even from the slightest bumps, children with epilepsy must not be excluded from social and recreational events due to fears of triggering convulsions. Some physicians feel that even boxing, wrestling, hockey, or football do not exacerbate seizure disorders but most doctors discourage rough contact sports because of the risk of head trauma.

Summer camps are great fun for children but not if they are excluded from athletic events, games, swimming, canoeing, and other activities. This can happen to children with epilepsy when parents have not had a thorough discussion with the camp counselor and have not agreed upon what can and what cannot be done. Crystal clear directions must be given in writing regarding the medications: what drugs to give, when and what to do in case of an emergency. Parents must never tire of educating others on epilepsy.

When a child with epilepsy is in camp, on trips, in various sports and social activities, or even at school, it is very helpful if they have a buddy who keeps a watchful eye, just in case of a seizure. This "buddy system" can be organized by parents, teachers, counselors, and even by the youngster with seizures.

Driving

Although driving is a necessity in our society, for teenagers it signifies independence, maturity, and adulthood. Accidents due to seizures are exceedingly rare in contrast to those caused by drunkenness. Yet, state regulations are more restrictive toward people with epilepsy than toward drinkers. In most states an individual with epilepsy cannot legally operate a motor vehicle unless a physician certifies that he or she has been seizure-free from 1 to 2 years and that from the medical point of view he or she is considered a safe driver.

The seizure-free period necessary for licensing depends on local laws and sometimes there are exceptions. For example, an individual with only night seizures may be allowed to drive or if the seizures occurred after treatment was discontinued, that person is allowed to drive as soon as the anticonvulsant drug in question is restarted. Some states have established an individual review on the basis of overall reliability and individual needs. It is the responsibility of the person who requests licensing to state truthfully whether he or she has epilepsy. Inquiries should be made at the Motor Vehicle Branches.

Many youngsters start taking their medication more conscientiously after they realize the necessity of having a seizure-free period for licensing. Parents should, ahead of time, discuss with their children the possibility of their not being able to operate a motor vehicle and when the seizures are still not fully controlled they should talk about "postponing" rather than "not being able" to drive.

Seventeen-year-old George Demchuk developed epilepsy following a head injury in a car accident in which his whole family was killed. He was raised by his aunt. During his seizures, usually lasting 10 to 15 seconds, he would stare unresponsively into space with his body somewhat rigid. Medications did not entirely abolish these attacks although his epilepsy did not inconvenience him too much.

George obtained his driver's license without the knowledge of his physician and he convinced his aunt to let him drive her car. A few weeks later, while driving on a busy downtown street, the friend who was with him noticed George staring into space, pressing the gas pedal, and speeding along. He hit an oncoming pickup truck; miraculously only his friend was hurt but not seriously.

George was held responsible by the police, not only for the accident but also for concealing his epilepsy when applying for a license. His license was withdrawn for a minimum of 1 year and until it could be proven through an official statement from his physician that his seizures were fully controlled.

Ralph Goodwin has been free of seizures for several years on anticonvulsant therapy. He had complex partial epilepsy but now only experiences the occasional initial warning feeling (aura) without having a complete seizure. He drove regularly. Whenever his aura slowly emerged he just stopped driving, or whatever he was doing, and usually in a minute the feeling was over. As time went on he became more lax with his medications.

One day at work, after his usual aura, Ralph did not recover but lost consciousness and had a full blown attack. He immediately notified his physician, took the bus to the clinic where a blood level of the anticonvulsant was obtained. It was low since Ralph had been rather lax in taking his pills. The low blood level explained his relapse. On the physician's advice he was allowed to drive but more frequent office visits were initiated.

Ralph did the right thing and followed the rules. He stopped driving, immediately notified his doctor who then investigated him and advised the special medical branch of the local Motor Vehicle Registry. Drivers with epilepsy should see their physicians regularly and follow the rules meticulously.

Parties, Alcohol, Pot, and Smoking

Many individuals with epilepsy have more seizures after irregular, disturbed nights and when they are overtired. For this reason, long parties reaching into the early morning hours, should be strictly avoided. Although alcohol is a drug with minimal anticonvulsant properties, it interacts with the metabolism of antiepileptic medications. In the case of Dilantin, for example, it lowers the blood level of that drug to what could be the breaking point in individuals with poorly controlled seizures. It may also cause excessive sedation when taken with certain anticonvulsants. Alcohol taken in moderation is generally permitted for those who are seizure-free on treatment, but excessive drinking is contraindicated. Even individuals without epilepsy may have convulsions following prolonged drinking bouts. (Figure 1).

Marijuana is not only illegal but its long-term effect on people with epilepsy is not fully known. On the other hand, hallucinogenic drugs frequently have longlasting disruptive effects on the functioning of the brain and may aggravate epilepsy. Smoking cigarettes, in the long run, is harmful to health. Those with uncontrolled epilepsy should smoke only when someone else is present because during an unexpected seizure a burning cigarette is a real fire hazard.

Dating and Marriage

One time, 5 years ago, my son asked his friends over for a small birthday party. One was a girl whom he loved madly. He had a seizure right in front of her and she ran home, 3 miles, terrified.

Dating is a time when all worrisome attitudes about epilepsy come into focus. It highlights such questions as Do I need to tell? What will people think if they find out? Who would want to marry a person with epilepsy?

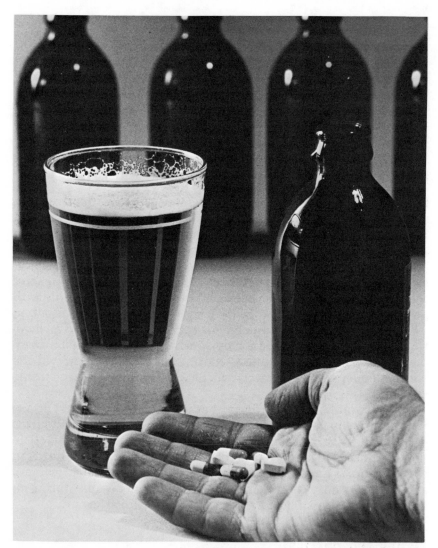

Figure 1.   The occasional social drink is permissible but heavy drinking, epilepsy, and
anticonvulsant medications do not mix.

Those with seizures should remember the importance of developing knowledge about epilepsy and being able to communicate that in appropriate situations. When individuals understand their form of seizures it is easier to share this information, at some point. Most dates are not total strangers. If the network of friends already knows, it is much easier to communicate; if not, "being found out" or "telling" presents a bigger worry. This problem has to be solved. Certainly, unless there is a very active form of epilepsy, the individual can decide if the date can be a good friend and when to tell. Friends need to form good attitudes, which is, of course, a gradual process. They should not just react because someone has epilepsy but look beyond at the qualities of the person. Prior to marriage, persons with epilepsy could arrange a discussion with their doctor and may request genetic counseling if necessary. (Also see the section on the hereditary aspects of epilepsy later in this chapter.)

Pregnancy

In recent years the number of teenage pregnancies have increased so dramatically that young unmarried girls have a 10% chance of getting pregnant. Younger teenagers are more at risk because they are less exposed to sex education and have more difficulty obtaining birth control devices.

Women with epilepsy must carefully plan their pregnancies and should request genetic counseling beforehand. Accidental pregnancy is even more traumatic when a chronic medical problem is present. Most seizure disorders are not hereditary, nevertheless, a potential mother needs to understand the risk of giving birth to a child who may develop seizures in later life. Some anticonvulsants decrease the effectiveness of birth control pills. More importantly, certain anticonvulsants such as Dilantin, Phenobarbital, especially heavy doses, can damage the developing fetus, mainly during the first few months of pregnancy (see Chapter 2). They may cause various birth defects or mental retardation. Malformations in the baby are more common when a combination of anticonvulsants are used in contrast to single therapy. In one study 23% of infants had birth defects when their mothers had received three or four drugs during pregnancy. Of course every drug, even aspirin and alcohol, may represent a potential danger to the fetus.

During pregnancy, careful medical monitoring is very important. In most cases treatment cannot be discontinued but certain drugs may be substituted prior to conception. For example, Dilantin could be replaced with Tegretol as it seems to be less toxic. As a general rule, the risk of seizures may increase during pregnancy because the anticonvulsant blood levels tend to fall particularly in the first trimester but this can be easily corrected by adjusting the dosage.

Occasionally a seizure-free state is maintained on less medication. Small seizures do not affect the fetus but prolonged and difficult convulsions may, besides being a potential danger to the mother. Again it needs to be emphasized that medications must never be stopped abruptly. Balancing the risk of damaging the fetus by severe convulsions or by anticonvulsants is a disturbing dilemma.

Breastfeeding

When nursing mothers are taking anticonvulsants their breastmilk also contains these medications. Although some of these substances may sedate the infant they have not been shown to be harmful. It is still helpful and reassuring for mothers to discuss breastfeeding with their physicians.

Is Epilepsy Hereditary? Genetic Counseling

In the past epilepsy was viewed strictly as an inherited condition. Children with seizures could not be adopted, many countries forbade the afflicted individuals to marry and a few regimes even sterilized them. Contrary to this old belief, recent studies show that most seizure disorders are acquired while a smaller proportion is inherited.

It is important to know whether epilepsy is hereditary, acquired, or both. Perhaps parents would like to have more children but will they also have epilepsy? What are the risks? Will these children pass this disorder on to their offsprings? What should relatives be told who also have or will have a family? If it is hereditary, from which side did it come? Men and women with epilepsy who are planning marriage must also know. Unfortunately, the answers to these important questions are often difficult because even highly trained epileptologists may find it hard to prove that some types of epilepsy are hereditary, acquired, or both. Hereditary factors can easily be ruled out when the cause of epilepsy is an abnormal pregnancy or birth, a tumor, meningitis, or a head injury. Many neurological diseases that are associated with seizures have a clear cut hereditary pattern. But how can a doctor help when there is no obvious cause for the seizures?

Certain epileptic disorders such as idiopathic generalized tonic-clonic convulsions, absence attacks (petit mal), photosensitive epilepsy, febrile, and some other types of seizures show a stronger hereditary pattern. The family history, the occurrence of the first seizure, the type of epilepsy, the neurological examination, certain EEG characteristics, and other tests all provide useful clues. On the basis of all this information, the specialist, who must be well-trained and experienced in epileptic disorders, can be more specific. Unfortunately, the genetic aspects of seizure disorders are very complex because the occurrence of epilepsy in an individual is due to many factors. These are age, sex, certain inherited tendencies, the presence, severity, and location of an injury, environmental influences, and even general health. For this reason the heredity of epilepsy is said to be multifactorial.

Surveys show that the rate of epilepsy in siblings is 5% when a child has any type of seizure, but 13% when it is generalized and the cause is unknown. Approximately 6% of children may develop seizures when one parent has idiopathic epilepsy. Mothers have a slightly higher chance of transmitting epileptic traits than fathers. If both parents have epilepsy the risk is 12%. These are generalizations but the previously described clues help the physician to be more specific.

Insurance

Individuals with epilepsy often pay higher automobile, health, and life insurance premiums. Recognizing that most persons with epilepsy are not poor insurance risks, the Epilepsy Foundation of America offers a Group Life Insurance Plan. Applications are processed through the Epilepsy Foundation of America, 1828 L Street, N.W., Washington, D.C. 20036.

Lay Epilepsy Organizations

Parents and their children with seizure disorders benefit greatly through exchanging their experiences with other families. To satisfy this need, in recent years hundreds of local lay epilepsy organizations were formed, meeting regularly. The importance for families to join such associations cannot be overemphasized; here they learn about services, other helpers, and facts about epilepsy. Parents realize their own strengths and weaknesses and most of all, that they are not alone. These organizations can also be a strong political force when legislative changes are needed.

After the diagnosis of epilepsy, parents could get in touch with another family who already have been "through the mill." Most of these parents are happy to listen, talk things over, and give advice because they know what it is like to be told that "your child has epilepsy"; they also recognize the need for joining lay epilepsy organizations.

The Rights of Children with Epilepsy
in Education, Employment, and Health

The rights of the handicapped were slow to be recognized. A right is something a person is entitled to and at the same time that someone else has to give. Public Law 94–142, the Education For All Handicapped Children Act is one of the most far reaching pieces of legislation affecting the handicapped, including those with epilepsy, in the United States. Canada has similar legislation. The Law became effective in September, 1977. It mandates free and appropriate education of handicapped children in the least restrictive environment. Consequently, children no longer are prevented from attending regular schools simply because they have epilepsy; their placement in special classes or separate schools is to occur only when their disabilities are such that education in regular classes, with the use of supplementary services, cannot be adequately met. The law has forced educators to better understand the disorder of epilepsy and it ensures an impartial hearing for parents who are not satisfied.

The Vocational Rehabilitation Act of 1973 and the Amendment of 1974 forbids the discrimination of the handicapped in hiring. Individuals who are otherwise qualified, cannot be excluded from a job solely because of their epilepsy. Any firm that receives more than $2,500 in funds and contracts per year from the Federal Government, must obey this law or risk loss of funding.

In 1973, The American Hospital Association published a "Patient's Bill of Rights," which has since received much publicity. Although it was mainly an effort to make the hospital staff more aware of the human needs of their patients, it is often promoted as a legal document and many states have enacted it as law. A hospital has many functions to perform including the prevention and treatment of disease, the education of professionals and patients and research. All these activities must be carried out with overriding concern for the patients (Annas, 1975; Rozovsky, 1980).

Communication with Helpers

The philosophy of rights is admirable but difficult to enforce because it deals mainly with human relationships. How can considerate and respectful health care be defined in legal terms? Laws cannot make teachers, employers, doctors, or nurses more friendly or more communicative, nor can they prevent a breakdown in personal relationships. Furthermore, there is a danger that the health staff (and this also applies to educators) instead of exercising their professional judgment in a humane manner will treat their patients only according to the rules. For example, when the parents insist on reading their child's records, they may in fact be confused by the medical terminology. Without detailed explanation and the willing cooperation of the physician, it is pointless for them to exercise their rights. Communication is so important that some medical centers, for example, the Comprehensive Epilepsy Program at the University of Minnesota, actively teach parents of children with seizures the best techniques in approaching and talking to professionals.

There are several reasons why it is difficult to communicate with health providers: limited time for discussions; doctors may be using technical language and not realizing that lay people do not understand it. There is still a myth that the physician's authority is unquestionable and many parents are too intimidated to ask questions. Some doctors are hesitant to answer because of their concern about upsetting the family or because of their inability to admit that nothing more can be done.

Parents need to come prepared to the physician's office with their thoughts well organized; they should decide beforehand what issues are important. The approach should be direct, honest, assertive, not overly aggressive, and respectful for the feelings and the rights of the doctor who is also a human being. When they do not understand something they should say so even if the physician has to repeat himself. Some individuals, after hearing the diagnosis or when treatment fails to control the seizures, direct their anger at the doctor rather than at the problem. While most physicians understand, aggressive behavior can only disrupt a mutual trusting relationship, and in the confrontation, the child is the loser.

In many epilepsy clinics nurses are taking on an expanded role. They are advocates of families, they teach parents and others about seizure disorders, make home and school visits, and even organize investigations. Although parents are often hesitant to ask questions from physicians they may eagerly talk about their concerns to nurses. During these exchanges much information emerges that may be extremely beneficial for both parties—the parents and their helpers. Nurse practitioners are invaluable members of a team of health professionals who now offer care to children with epilepsy.

Parents must not be afraid to tell health providers about their concerns. They should remember that they pay for these services and also, that the vast majority of health professionals are dedicated people who want to help.

Suggested Reading

Annas, G. J., 1975. The Rights of Hospital Patients, Avon, New York.
Rozovsky, L. E., 1980. The Canadian Patient's Book of Rights. Doubleday, Toronto.

chapter 13

The Multihandicapped

The Burden of a Multihandicapped Child

Most Handicaps Are Not Readily Apparent at Birth

The Team Approach

Labels

Learning Difficulties

Hyperactivity

Mental Retardation

Cerebral Palsy

Visual and Hearing Impairment,
  Speech and Language Delay

Behavioral Problems

How to Use Limits to Help Children Grow and Learn

References

Often it is very difficult for the parents to cope with the problems of their multihandicapped child. The purpose of this chapter is not to describe in detail all handicaps but to offer some general suggestions and selected references so parents can more easily obtain further information.

The Burden of a Multihandicapped Child

Roy Williams, a 13-year-old, tall, multihandicapped boy, was referred by his school nurse for better seizure control. He was attending a special school for retarded children but lived at home. Roy had marked mental retardation. The right side of his body was weak due to a birth injury and he had frequent convulsions. He was still not fully toilet trained.

During the physical examination it immediately became clear that Roy, who had to be coaxed a great deal, was difficult to handle. Suddenly, without warning, he flung out his arms, hitting his mother's shoulder quite hard; she tried to minimize this painful and somewhat embarrassing incident. One could not help wondering how the parents had managed to live with this severely handicapped boy. How did they raise two other children and yet survive? When the parents were asked if they had ever considered institutionalization they answered, "yes, but we decided against it." "Well, how did you cope all these years?" "Doctor, it was hell, but we love him!"

Roy's convulsions could not be controlled in spite of major changes in his medications. Doctors could offer no more and this was freely discussed with the parents. Nevertheless, they were asked to make an appointment with the social worker. Mr. and Mrs. Williams had not gone out together for a social evening for over 10 years because babysitters could not handle Roy. After his convulsions he was irritable and often scratched, bit, and hit out at people. The social worker proposed the use of once a week volunteer babysitting service which was available only for parents of handicapped children. The social worker also discussed cheaper ways of obtaining the anticonvulsant medications, certain tax benefits for families of handicapped children, and suggested that the parents join a parent association of the mentally retarded. Finally she pointed out that after the age of 18, Roy might be able to go to a government operated group home for the severely handicapped. She suggested the parents put his name on the waiting list. This was the greatest relief

189

for the parents who looked upon their own retirement with insecurity. They would not be able to ask their other children to look after Roy but at the same time realized that they themselves would no longer be able to cope.

Then the parents visited a residential school for the retarded. They learned that Roy could go home during weekends and that enrollment into this program did not mean final institutionalization. Still the parents declined to admit their son but on learning about the special summer camp program they decided to put him into that facility for 6 weeks. This would allow the family to have their first holiday together in 10 years. Families of multihandicapped children can be helped in many ways!

Looking after a multihandicapped child can be an enormous burden on the family. It means greatly increased expenses, more work for the parents, less recreation, less time for the other children and for each other. Physicians can only do so much.

Nevertheless, the family can be helped. First, the parents must understand the abilities and weaknesses of their multihandicapped children in order to meet their developmental needs. Therefore, one or more detailed multi-disciplinary evaluations are necessary. Next, they must choose and organize the best available services. Here they may require help from an experienced social worker, community health nurse, or counselors. This is because these services are complex and vary from place to place and because the need of one particular child may be special. Finally, the needs of every family member must be taken into consideration (Chapter 11). Parents should not be too proud or too shy to ask for help, and they must plan ahead.

Most Handicaps Are Not Readily Apparent at Birth

The incidence of additional handicaps is higher in children with epilepsy because when the brain has one malfunction, there is more of a chance for another. Thus learning difficulties, mental retardation, speech and language delay, cerebral palsy, poor coordination, and visual and hearing impairments are more common.

Most chronic handicaps are not readily apparent at birth. The daily reflex functioning of an infant is controlled by the lower brain structures rather than the cortex or hemispheres, which are responsible for complex behavior. With age the hemispheres mature and take over this control while the primitive reflex behavior gradually disappears. When the higher cortical centers are damaged, initially the problems, if at all apparent, are subtle but they become more and more marked with age. For this reason the developmental evaluation of a 6-month-old may still be inaccurate whereas, that of a 5-year-old child is more definitive. Although the experienced physician may discover or predict seemingly hidden problems in the early months of life, chronic handicaps are usually diagnosed later. An early diagnosis is crucially important because precious time should not be wasted without appropriate treatment.

The Team Approach

Treating only the seizures is inadequate and may even be unsuccessful when the child has other handicaps.

> Brian Hatford had poorly controlled temporal lobe epilepsy and a severe learning disability. They both caused considerable stress. The child's physician, after many trials, felt that medications alone would not stop the seizures unless the pressures at school were removed. This led to a detailed psychological evaluation and significant changes in Brian's education. As soon as the pressures subsided the seizure control dramatically improved.

As medical knowledge mushroomed during this century, a single physician could no longer deal adequately with all aspects of health care and, therefore, more and more specialization has taken place. In most cases though, the family doctor or pediatrician together with the parents, can look after a child's medical problems; referral to a more specialized physician is seldom necessary. But when the child is multihandicapped, this system can be cumbersome, time consuming, and ineffective.

> Vivian, who was 4 years old, had epilepsy, cerebral palsy, speech delay, and a moderate hearing loss. Her family had just arrived in the city because the father had been promoted to a new job. Although Vivian had had numerous evaluations in her early childhood, she needed a reassessment and her treatment had to be reorganized. The parents selected a local family physician who made several referrals to different specialists. One by one they saw Vivian (after considerable waiting time for appointments) and they recommended further evaluations in different parts of the city, such as, x-rays, EEG, blood tests, hearing assessment, and a visit to a speech pathologist and to a hospital physiotherapist. This took more time. Each health professional advised them only in his own area and since the doctors did not have contact with one another, some of their recommendations conflicted. The parents were confused. As treatment began the mother took Vivian to the hospital three times for physiotherapy and twice a week to a medical building several miles away for speech therapy; this meant taking Vivian out of her preschool program and proved so unsatisfactory that the child was referred to an evaluation clinic. After a 2-day-long evaluation the child

was enrolled into their special preschool program where physiotherapy and speech therapy were also provided. This type of multi-disciplinary treatment approach was a much happier arrangement.

In an attempt to improve the care of the multihandicapped, the team approach has been introduced. It is not the family who goes to the specialists located in various parts of the city but the specialists who come to the child, so to speak; they see the child in a medical clinic where he or she has been brought for an evaluation. This is carried out by the many different professionals and in most cases can be completed in a couple of days. The parents do not receive conflicting opinions and generally do not "shop around" for advice. The assessment is more accurate because the team members all become familiar with the child and through interaction they reinforce one another's findings. Also, the treatment for the multihandicapped child is more organized.

Labels

A child's neurological problems depend on what parts of the brain are affected and how severely. The coordination can be so mildly abnormal that it is simply called clumsiness. It may be that due to a severe birth injury the child cannot speak, walk, or swallow; in this case he or she is said to have marked cerebral palsy. At the same time, the manifestations of cerebral palsy may be so minimal that the abnormal neurological signs are hardly noticeable. Most physicians are reluctant to diagnose mental retardation in young children unless it is very obvious. When the delay is minimal or specific to one area, it may be referred to as a developmental delay and this can be a motor, mental, speech, or a language lag. While the term *lag* suggests that the child will catch up, this is not always so. Growth and development may be slower because of normal individual variations, lack of opportunities to learn skills, as in the case of a child who is neglected, or due to various neurological reasons. Brain damage simply indicates that at one stage in the child's life the brain sustained some type of injury. This is perhaps the most frightening label to the parents who may incorrectly think that such an individual is not capable of learning. Minimal brain dysfunction is also a commonly used term. It implies that due to different causes the brain malfunctions minimally. Therefore, such a child can be inattentive, overactive, clumsy, with or without minimal speech, learning and behavior problems. The neurological examination or subsequent investigations may show subtle abnormalities.

Parents must remember that medical labels do not always have practical significance. Many diagnostic terms "label" children sometimes for years and for this reason they are often disliked. Although labels are often needed to obtain appropriate services, they might also limit the expectations for a child and therefore be damaging. Nevertheless, they are widely used.

Learning Difficulties

Learning difficulties are common in children with epilepsy. There are three main reasons for this: brain dysfunction may be present in addition to epilepsy, occasionally frequent or prolonged seizures interfere with learning, and medications may make the child tired, sleepy, and less alert.

Learning is a complex, physiological task. Because during learning children rely on much of their brain, ("a marvelous computer") even subtle malfunctions here and there may disturb their receptive and expressive language, reading, writing, spelling, arithmetic, short- and long-term memory, visual or auditory perception, fine motor coordination and many other necessary skills. In many families, due to complex genetic inheritance, learning disabilities are passed down from generation to generation, mainly along the male side. At other times, the development of the brain, which consists of billions of cells and intricate pathways, is impaired. Finally, brain damage may have occurred during pregnancy, at birth, or after. When possible, the term *brain damage* should be avoided because people, including some educators, frequently believe that children with brain damage cannot learn. This is, of course, not true.

The best way to manage children with a learning disability is to obtain a careful psychoeducational evaluation that pinpoints their strengths and weaknesses. Then an appropriate remedial teaching curriculum can be designed to fit their needs. A thorough evaluation and a good teacher in a suitable class are the keys to successful remedial teaching. An excellent book on this subject is available for the parents (Smith, 1981).

Seizures often interfere with the process of learning. A child with petit mal may have hundreds of attacks within 1 hour, with each seizure interrupting his or her thinking. Petit mal epilepsy can be so subtle that not infrequently these children are thought to be lazy because they cannot finish their work in time, inattentive because they miss the teacher's instructions, disruptive because they may ask questions at the wrong time, or just plain dumb. Other types of seizures cause tiredness and lethargy so the entire day may be ruined. These children often have good and bad days.

> Frank Porter had frequent early morning seizures—usually around 6 or 7 o'clock in the morning—in his bed. Initially the parents did not observe them, and Frank did not recall the events so for a while no one realized he had epilepsy. Due to his seizures, there were many days when for no apparent reason he was waking up with great difficulty and he felt extremely tired, sometimes for the whole day. He was just not able to study. After his seizures were discovered and treated he no longer had problems in school.

Heavy medications can slow down learning. Barbiturates, such as phenobarbital and Mysoline, may produce sleepiness, tiredness, restlessness, and poor concentration, in which case they may need to be replaced with another anticonvulsant. It is possible that many other drugs also interfere with the child's behavior and learning in subtle ways. Therefore, the selection of the medications and the dose given are crucial decisions. In order to keep the child fully alert it is often helpful if the heavier doses are given at night rather than in the morning or during the day.

Parents should carefully watch the progress of their child with epilepsy and when the medication seems to interfere with learning, they should not hesitate to discuss this with their physician. The aim of good seizure management is to have happy, healthy, and seizure-free children who are able to utilize the full extent of their abilities.

Hyperactivity

Although hyperactive children have always been around, in recent years they have received much attention from many different professionals. In a strict sense, hyperactivity is not a diagnosis but a description of behavior. Typically, these children cannot concentrate, they fidget constantly, they are in constant motion, and they may have low frustration tolerance, poor coordination, learning disability, and they may be irritable. Studies have shown that about half of all children are described as overactive by their parents or teachers at one time or another. Many such children are restless and learn poorly in school but show no such behavior at home where the expectations are different. The management is not always easy and the parents may need professional help. Children with epilepsy are occasionally hyperactive, often due to medications. A number of informative books were written for parents on this subject (Stewart and Olds, 1973; Safer and Allen, 1976).

Mental Retardation

The usual definition of mental retardation is an IQ (intelligence quotient) of 70 or less. The incidence of 3% is the most commonly quoted figure for the proportion of retarded individuals in the general population but it is higher when epilepsy is present. The IQ range from 50 to 70 is often referred to as "educable mental retardation," and those in the 30 to 50 range are called "trainable." Trainable implies that these children are less likely to learn school subjects. The public image of mentally retarded persons—a person who is helpless or who cannot develop self-care skills and who learns nothing—is not an accurate one. It is especially important for parents to know that many mentally retarded persons can become productive members of society with special assistance. Again, it has to be emphasized that epilepsy does not lead to mental retardation but rather these two are the result of a disorder in the brain.

The diagnosis of subnormality has major implications for that child and the family; therefore, it should be ascertained only through a careful evaluation. Realistic acceptance of the condition is important because mentally retarded children develop at their own rate and greatly benefit from being exposed to rich learning experiences in the appropriate environment (Bernard and Powell, 1972).

Cerebral Palsy

By definition, cerebral palsy is a motor disability due to brain damage, before, during, or shortly after birth. It may be minimal or severe. The body and limbs of these children may be stiff, limp, tremulous, unsteady, always poorly coordinated, and may show involuntary movements, or a mixture of all of these. It is not a progressive disorder and not an illness. Because children with cerebral palsy tend to be multihandicapped, a multidisciplinary approach to the diagnosis and treatment is important. Physical and occupational therapy and orthopedic surgery are particularly helpful in their treatment. In most major medical centers cerebral palsy clinics exist where all these services are provided and coordinated. Each child must be handled on an individual basis. The prevalence of cerebral palsy in the general population is one to two per thousand. A useful book for parents is given in the References (Finnie, 1975).

Visual and Hearing Impairment, Speech and Language Delay

Impaired vision has enormous implications for that individual. Children with total blindness do not develop spontaneously and every skill has to be taught to them. Even those with partial vision must receive specialized help, mainly during their school years. Approximately 10 to 15 percent of legally blind children have epilepsy. This is a large and complex area but fortunately a network of services and informative books are available for parents (Scott, Jan, and Freeman, 1977).

Hearing loss is a "hidden" handicap that can significantly influence the life of a child. The most comprehensive book for parents is by Freeman, Carbin, and Boose (1981). Speech disturbance and language delay are also common handicaps but can be improved with professional help (Schreiber, 1973).

There are other additional disabilities such as heart disease, cleft palate, and orthopedic problems that may affect children with epilepsy, but these are not discussed.

Behavioral Problems

The increased occurrence of behavioral disorders in children with epilepsy has been extensively studied. Epilepsy is a symptom of an underlying disturbance in the mechanisms of the brain. The same disturbance may also affect the way specific parts of the brain function. This then can account for disorders of learning or attention or the modulation of feelings that contribute to emotional difficulties. For example, when children with epilepsy cannot attend well (without being distracted) they may have trouble responding when called. If sent to get a spoon, on the way to the kitchen they wind up playing with a toy noticed in the hall. Parental frustration mounts when these events occur 100 times a day (instead of just 30 times). Angry exchanges, back and forth, can develop and this may only lead to further behavioral deterioration.

Language is used to define, categorize, and organize situations. When receptive (understanding) or expressive (the use of) language is affected, these children carry out the wrong instruction or are unable to explain that they disagree or don't understand, and therefore, are apt to get confused and frustrated. Sometimes, even more subtle disorders of brain function cause behavioral problems.

As evident from the above discussions, children with epilepsy are more vulnerable to difficulties when they are acquiring many different skills and also when they are learning how to control their behavior and interaction. How parents help themselves and their children to compensate for these weaknesses depends a great deal on their understanding of the children and on how they interact with them at home. Some individuals have difficulty mastering the complex routines of social interaction or modulating their moods.

In remedial teaching, the reading process of slow learners is broken down, simplified, and then taught. Similarly the steps of social interaction must be tailored to the needs of children with behavior problems. These youngsters will always be disadvantaged in the peer culture where the sequences of interaction are scattered, at times capricious, and subject to arbitrary power. They may be seen as aggressive, impulsive, and inconsistent.

Due to this vulnerability, clear rules are very important and these should be respectively reinforced with verbal encouragement and occasional concrete rewards. Furthermore, their environment must be structured because they tend to react to the unusual, unpredicted event (although perhaps predictable to our eyes) with an impulsive or poorly chosen action. When the steps of a social interaction are gone awry, each time it will be necessary for the parents to review them with the child in a calm fashion. Although this can be tiresome and frustrating it is the best way to prevent additional psychological problems, family distress and further peer alienation. Because of this increased stress on the family, therapists with knowledge of child management techniques and family skills will often be valuable assistants.

When children with seizures and other handicaps have behavioral difficulties, both the child and the family are heavily taxed. Therefore, psychological reactions may occur. Helpers with various skills are often required to pool their expertise in order to define the different aspects of a problem and to lay out some beneficial steps. As previously discussed, this type of interdisciplinary team approach is the best possible way to deal with difficult complex situations.

How to Use Limits to Help Children Grow and Learn

The Basic Principles

What is a limit? It is a guideline for behavior that should be defined clearly and briefly. Limits are only useful if children know by the attitudes of their parents that they believe in them and enforce them. Reasonable consequences must also be clearly stated should these rules be broken. Whenever possible, rules should be the same for both children and adults. For example, it is harder to teach a child not to swear if bad language is often used in the home by the parents.

Why are limits important? Children need to feel safe from their own impulses. When they get angry or are frustrated, their natural response may be to throw things or to hit someone. They must learn that they can experience these feelings without being destructive. Rather than acting out they can say, "I am mad" or "that is hard to do! I hate it!"

Rules are also important in developing a sense of responsibility. Children learn that what they do has consequences and when they begin to experience different feelings they learn to make choices about what to do. They can stop and think. Through the use of rules and limits they will take other people's feelings into account. For example, when one child calls another a "dummy" it is possible to offer a correction. "I know you are mad at Sally but calling her a dummy hurts her. You don't like to be called a dummy. Let's tell her what you are mad about and see if we can figure out what to do." Here, a rule is combined with problem solving. Both are needed. Many times only the rule, "don't call people names" may be used but it is important for a child to have an opportunity for alternative problem solving.

Limits should be brief and few in number. Children cannot remember too many rules. Those with learning disabilities or who are impulsive have an even harder time because it is more difficult for them to understand and remember. Memories can be strengthened by parents who compliment the children when they "stop and think" and remember the rules. Limits create an atmosphere of safety and respect. Knowing that others also follow the rules allows children to explore the intriguing aspects of the world that attracts them. Their respect for others will help people admire and encourage them.

Which rules are most important? Some rules are necessary for the safety of the child and others (this should always be explained). Some are important for the development of respect for people—even preschoolers can understand the golden rule: "Do unto others as you would have others do unto you."

Limits are needed to protect property and also the sanity of parents. The shrieking of children makes some parents very upset while it does not bother others. Still it is important to expect children to respect their parents' needs (and vice versa) so that the mutual caring that is required can flourish.

Practical Suggestions about Rules

Is the limit enforceable? Can the child learn that when a rule is broken, a consequence will be imposed if the parents find out? For example, the rule of never using certain words may not be enforceable as most children occasionally swear with their peer groups and in moments of frustration (just like adults).

Is it possible to provide additional clues about the rule? Most children cannot remember even a few rules all the time. When parents are with their children in an aggravating situation, calling their names or raising an eyebrow can remind them to stop and think. Visual or auditory clues can be helpful to keep rules working well for the child, such as a rope at the end of a driveway to limit bike riding or a whistle.

How long are limits necessary? Rules should be reviewed periodically to make most sense for the age and nature of children. Some require continued restrictions about their access to a store or refrigerator while others can enjoy these newly acquired privileges earlier because of their responsible behavior. Rules need to be lifted periodically (except when safety is involved) to see if the child can handle a new responsibility. There is a higher risk of error in a new opportunity but it can be a learning situation that need not result in the replacement of the old rule. For example, if a child is given permission to cook his own chocolate milk on the stove, it may boil over. The parent will have a mess to clean up with him but also a chance to say, "stoves can be dangerous and that is why you were not allowed to use it before. Now, you know that you have to keep watching and thinking to avoid an accident."

Is that limit mainly for the convenience of the adults? If parents think only about their own convenience and do not consider the children, there could be two thousand rules—children are rarely convenient.

Does the rule interfere with more constructive activities or experimenting with more grown up behavior? Just saying, "don't talk to strangers" or "don't play with Alice's toys" can limit a child's world of experience. Of course, some kids are very destructive with the toys of others and so limiting rules may be necessary; as far as talking to strangers is concerned, safe opportunities can be provided to enrich the child's experiences.

Is the limit reinforced in other settings? Parents should create consistency, as much as possible, in the child's world. Relatives, close friends, teachers, and babysitters should know the rules in the family and the words used to teach them. The greater the child's behavioral difficulty, the more important is the consistency in all aspects of the environment as well as repetitive communication.

Should the punishment fit the crime? Yes. Consequences must be a logical outcome of the misbehavior or violation of the rule. For example, taking someone else's toy without permission should result in the loss of its use for a period of time. Hitting (after the problem is understood and discussed) can lead to a "time out." After breaking something the child should do some chores to help pay for it. If a child fails to put away a game, it can be "off-limits" for a day. Obviously, following up on these consequences takes a lot of time and effort.

Enforcement of Rules

Limits must be kept consistently. Children like to test their parents, therefore, limits should be consistent. When a rule has been erratically reinforced, it takes much longer to get it working well again.

Children naturally test limits. Children believe actions more than words. They like to see that what parents say is what they do. This applies to both positive and negative statements. If it seems that a rule or a promise is not likely to be reinforced, it is better to hold one's tongue.

The fewer rules that are created, the easier it is. Rules must be important to parents, necessary for the safety of the child and for the creation of mutual respect. Rules need to be mentioned hundreds of times in one form or another during the growth and development of a child and even more for the congenitally or behaviorally handicapped. Therefore, the fewer the rules, the easier it is for parents to keep their word.

Steps in Setting Limits

Discuss the rules. At neutral times, children should be told the whys and wherefores of the family's rules. Limits do not need to be changed just because they resent it. Their feelings should be considered, however, as the restriction is again reviewed.

Rules should be restated when the need arises. Parents should be clear and brief. They need to call their child's name with a firm but pleasant voice. For example, "Jeffrey, I don't want you to hit your sister!" or "Lisa, you are not allowed to play with the stove." If possible, problem solving should be used: "Jeffrey, come draw with your crayons now" or "Lisa, we can cook something together tomorrow."

The warning. If the behavior persists, children need to be reminded of the rules and consequences. Now if they repeat it again, it has been done with the knowledge that it can lead to punishment. For example, "Jeffrey, I told you not to hit your sister. If you hit her again, you will have a time-out." (Five minutes sitting alone in a designated spot away from favorite games or social activities.) Time-out for longer than 5 minutes has no increased effect and should be avoided. Such a procedure can be as simple as pulling a child's chair away from the lunch table for a couple of minutes, then allowing him or her to return.

Enforcement. Parents must follow through with the consequences they warned about. When the punishment is finished, they should treat their children as if nothing had happened. The penalty has been paid and they are entitled to another chance.

The rules probably will not have to be restated now. Most young children will remember the limits for a day or so (if there are not too many) and school-age youngsters will remember for about a week (if there are no developmental problems). Should Jeffrey hit his sister tomorrow, then he can again be given the warning before the punishment is enforced. The parents may find *How to Discipline with Love* by Dodson (1978) a good, informative book.

References

Bernard, K. E., and Powell, M. L. 1972. Teaching The Mentally Retarded Child. A family care approach. C. V. Mosby, St. Louis.

Dodson, F. 1978. How To Discipline With Love. New American Library/ Signet Book, New York.

Finnie, N. R. 1975. Handling The Young Cerebral Palsied Child At Home, Second Edition. E. P. Dutton, New York.

Freeman, R. D., Carbin, C. F., and Boose, R. J. 1981. Can't Your Child Hear? University Park Press, Baltimore.

Safer, D. J., and Allen, R. P. 1976. Hyperactive Children. Diagnosis and Management. University Park Press, Baltimore.

Schreiber, F. R. 1973. Your Child's Speech. Hash-Marc/Ballantine Books, New York.

Scott, E. P., Jan, J. E., and Freeman, R. D. 1977. Can't Your Child See? University Park Press, Baltimore.

Smith, S. L. 1981. No Easy Answers: The Learning Disabled Child. Bantam Books, New York.

Stewart, M. A., and Olds, S. W. 1973. Raising A Hyperactive Child. Harper and Row, New York.

chapter 14

Preparation for Work and Employment

J. Lynne Mann, M.A., A.R.W., Clinical and Rehabilitation Psychologist

Early Childhood
Elementary School Years
Transition to Secondary School
Secondary School Years
Preparation for the Job Hunt
Maintaining and Moving Up in Jobs
Summary of the Career Development Process

Adults with epilepsy often state that employment is one of their most pressing concerns. Discrimination is cited as the main reason for the difficult time they have in finding work that is satisfying, but clearly there are other causes.

> Frank Roberts, a 23-year-old man who was referred for vocational counseling, stated that he had experienced discrimination at job interviews so often that he had stopped applying. Referral information disclosed that he had complex partial seizures, long-standing difficulty in getting along with others and in managing his own life separately from helpers. Communication with a job finding organization indicated that he had been offered several job opportunities, all of which he had turned down. Frank wanted to work only as a logger and this was an impossible goal. He would not consider any other possible jobs even though he was having frequent major convulsions. Many employers had told him they would not hire him because of the possible dangers which might result.

Was this a case of discrimination? Perhaps, but several other questions also had to be considered. Was this discrimination or true concern for his safety on the employer's part? Was his lack of realistic planning limiting his employment possibilities? What kinds of attitudes toward employers and others did he have, which might have affected his planning abilities or his job interviews? Was this person experiencing adjustment difficulties? How much career exploration had occurred before his referral? Were his intellectual abilities affecting his ability to reason out a new course of action?

This chapter explores these questions and offers suggestions that will help children in planning their career realistically with their parents' assistance.

The single most important fact to grasp about planning for future employment is that career preparation is a developmental process. Much as infants progress from total dependence to adulthood and beyond in tiny steps, so does career/job awareness, education, exploration, and try-out occur in a sequence. Steps that are missed or rushed create stumbling blocks later on in the process.

Early Childhood

People, whether or not they have epilepsy, begin preparing themselves or are being prepared for work as young children, even before kindergarten. Usually, that preparation occurs naturally, in the context of the family first and then with playmates. Most of this early learning is nonspecific and lies within the area of attitudes about the world of work. Much of this exposure happens around the dinner table:

Ron: *What happened with you today Marge?*

Marge: *Don't ask! I was late getting there because the parking lot was full again. My boss handed me seven reports that she wanted done before noon. I had lunch with that guy from the Sales Department that I told you about and I seemed to be on the run all afternoon.*

Ron: *Sorry I asked. Can I have more meat?*

The young child listening probably won't remember or even understand a lot of this conversation but will get an impression that today was not mom's greatest day ever. On other days the child may sense that work is exciting, challenging, and rewarding but hard. Out of this table-talk, a general impression emerges about the value and purpose of work. Parents should be aware of the importance of these table conversations for the later career maturity of their children. They must not restrict their discussions to only the wonderful parts of working. Much of it is not fascinating or rewarding but we all live with that reality. Some of us do so more effectively than others because our attitudes and expectations are not unrealistic.

During their preschool years children spend a great deal of time playing out fantasies. They dress up like mom and dad, buy and sell, play school, they become cowboys, firemen, pilots, doctors, nurses, and superman or spiderman. This is not only great fun but also a wonderful opportunity to learn about different roles and jobs. They gain experience by seeing their parents' place of work. By the time they enter kindergarten most can tell us about some specific types of jobs that are possible. They are already beginning to learn that work means many different things. There are workers called mothers, doctors, nurses, farmers, teachers, police officers, Santa Claus, elves, firemen, and maybe storekeepers, newsboys, and bosses. Parents can point out these jobs to their children when it seems a natural extension of conversation.

Parents of a child with epilepsy may make many trips back and forth to the doctor's office or hospital clinic. It's a possibility that the child may begin to see the work world as full of medical helpers. Childhood is a time for fantasy about jobs, so if a youngster first says he or she is going to be a doctor, there is no need to set up a college fund. Some parts of this job that might be appealing could be acknowledged and discussed. The parents are beginning to stimulate their child's problem-solving or decision-making skills at the level of a fun conversation. They can use the bus ride or car ride to and from the office for pointing out other occupations. At this time, the main career/job preparation task is informal exposure and education. A formal description of a policeman's duties, as an example, will be boring.

Elementary School Years

Starting school is a significant job awareness event. This is easily overlooked because it is also, and more importantly, the first giant step away from the known world. Up until this time, children have grown used to seeing the family for most of the daytime hours and only a few nursery school teachers or babysitters. Suddenly there are other adults and children, new buildings and a distance between them and their old environment. At school they will be meeting teachers, principals, teachers' aides, a nurse, and perhaps helpers at the playground. If they have special learning needs, there may also be a psychologist, a tutor or counselor. All of these people belong to a special group of workers: they are helpers.

The school may already have a career awareness program. It could be part of a social studies or a civics class or it may consist of occasional field trips to places of employment. Factories are often chosen because their products are so highly visible.

Teachers stress the relationship between present study habits or classroom behavior and future job expectations . . . "it's really important to be on time for class, just like your mom and dad have to be on time for their jobs. Going to school is your job for the next few years." They may give assignments to students to name the chores they are already doing at home, which ones they enjoy or would like to learn how to do. The process of career development becomes slightly more formal in that teachers begin to explore the student's interests, skills, dreams, or fantasies. This is still much too early to expect choices to be made; mainly education and fantasy are stressed.

No doubt, parents will hear: "Mommy, Miss Jones is wonderful, she's so smart and she knows way more than you and dad and I'm going to be a teacher just like her when I grow up. . . Mr. Jenkins said I could stay after school tomorrow and help him sweep the gym; isn't that great, dad?" Encouragement and interest are as important now as always. But, what if parents are beginning to worry that their children are getting their hopes up too high? Will they be headed for a large disappointment in a few years when they find out that being a teacher means having to complete several years of college? Or what if parents are afraid about the reaction of relative strangers to the seizures in class? People at school may be having similar fears of hurting the feelings of students with epilepsy. Will they restrict the children's chances for learning about work by stifling what seems to them to be "wild dreams" about jobs? Will they restrict them from after school activities?

Parents may be in the midst of learning to cope with their own fears and doubts about their children's future. Still they may be asked by the principal to speak about epilepsy in a manner that will relieve the teacher's concerns and allow them to offer a variety of opportunities and new experiences. Parents may even need to speak to the classmates explaining, at their level of understanding, what a seizure is. The alternative is that students with epilepsy may be given more concessions than others just because they have epilepsy. This specialized treatment, where unwarranted, creates an expectation for future allowances to be made outside school, perhaps in the work world.

> Paul Cronin, a 24-year-old man had come through a special program in his local school. Educationally, his classes had always been ungraded and his marks were referred to as "compassionate" grades. He progressed to a specialized waiter training program at his community college. He then decided it was time to look for work. His seizures were well controlled. He located a job as a kitchen helper. Feeling pleased with his efforts, he began his employment only to quit next day because "they" expected him to work "way too hard." He compared the expectations for work to those of his former teachers and found them terribly unjust.

In a sense, this young man had been led down a cruel garden path by caring individuals who had considered his self-concept needs but not his need for effective planning or decision making skills. Parents will meet these well-intentioned people who under-prepare or over-expect. It will be their added responsibility to restore a sense of balance to these individuals who are reacting out of their lack of understanding of what epilepsy means.

The above described school experiences teach the responsibilities of adult workers/students. The pamphlets written by the Epilepsy Foundation of America for school personnel and classmates will also be of great assistance in teaching them about seizures. When parents look toward the future of their children as adult workers this will help others to achieve a sense of balance as they work with the students. Effective career planning, whenever it occurs, takes into account:

Self-actualization
Self-esteem
Love and belonging
Safety
Physiological needs

Those students who have lost sight of the everyday world's expectations for work well done (or done adequately) and not for work that was a "good effort" will have to learn this later. Actually many young adults, those with epilepsy included, are having to take courses in proper work habits or proper work attitudes.

In the elementary school years the child acquires good or poor work habits both in school and at home as well. Some children learn that their safety needs not only have priority over their other requirements but may also exclude them as important

> David's mother, came to see a counselor for assistance in dealing with the child's recently developed "stubbornness." She states: "It seems that lately every time I ask him to clean up his toys or his room, he ignores me. If I push it by nagging at him he has even said things like: "If you make me do it, I'm gonna have a seizure."

Much can be said about this interchange but clearly, David has learned that his epilepsy is more important than his human responsibilities to others. Is this so dissimilar from the employee who comes in late repeatedly because he was too tired to get up?

Transition to Secondary School

Very important decisions for future vocational choices occur in the seventh and eighth grades. The student with epilepsy, who has no associated learning difficulties, will almost automatically proceed from an academically oriented junior high program to an academically oriented secondary program. The student who is a special needs learner may have the option to enter a prevocationally oriented secondary school. Alternately, the secondary school program may continue to be classroom based curriculums with the subjects becoming geared to increasing independent living skills.

At this age, the school personnel will not make such an important decision based only on the students' opinions of what would be their preferred path. Careful planning with all concerned needs to occur. By this time the parents will have a fairly reliable idea of their children's best learning environment. If they have always learned best by exploring or touching objects, by manipulating toys to figure out how they work (and how to break them), these are the children who will benefit most from a secondary school program that involves "hands-on" experiences. In the special area of career planning, a school program that includes a work education and experience component might be excellent to advocate for the child. Some work education/experience programs (WEP) consist of two field trips per semester, some WEP coordinators find half-day per week semester blocks of work experience, some can arrange two or more full days per week to be spent in work sites trying out jobs that a student thinks might be interesting. Should such programs exist in the school district, the students will be able to explore the fantasies they have been thinking about for years. Awareness of what a job means, of what it can involve, builds, and so exploration becomes another step in the career development process available within the school setting. Exploration may already have begun at home if the child volunteers his labor around the neighborhood, or has a part-time weekend job.

The child with epilepsy may be an average or above average student. There are still good reasons to wish for a WEP component to be planned in these transition years. For example, if that child has had a long and hard time achieving maximal seizure control then some of the side effects of this may have been reduced exposure to the world of making friends, getting around town independently, fear of trying things alone, or a generally lowered positive self-concept. These WEP programs have a characteristically positive effect on such adjustment difficulties, particularly where they have been running for some time with many work sites well-established.

These years can be transitional in another manner. Some students with epilepsy may have been placed in special education classes during elementary school. And later, they must be reintegrated into regular classes. Again the parents' advocacy will be important along with the planning efforts of the school.

Secondary School Years

In the last 3 to 4 years of public school, students will plan the "what next" phase. Their need to see ahead as well as that of others involved in their lives will crystalize. Fantasy and their early awareness about the world of work are no longer sufficient as the time comes to leave school and as adulthood approaches. Their school programs may be preparing them to make some initial career decisions through commercial science/business courses, work experience programs, career days and trips into industry. Or, the continued academics may be the focus. The children, generally, go through a period of self-analysis. This means evaluating what kind of an individual they are and what they can do. Some of the important aspects of career development at this time are: assessing interests, hobbies, job or job-related skills, planning and organizing abilities and comparing oneself to known employed persons.

In assisting a child-soon-to-become-adult, the fantasy jobs ("I'm going to be a race-car driver, dad") do not need to be formally shelved. Help may be needed, however, in picking through and pulling out the usable parts ("it sounds like you still have a strong interest in what makes cars and machines work well").

Having defined an interest, a young person must investigate how it can be used in different jobs. Most state employment agencies have information on this. The school may arrange for graduating students to visit these offices. Here, facts are available about measuring or evaluating the requirements of a job or job group, about the availability of employment in geographic areas and about the various training routes in entering the work world. Most school counselors are also well-informed.

The positive outcome of this stage in the development process is movement from fantasy, through awareness and exploration to tentative commitment. That is, the child's final decision about "what next" is not final at all; it is only the first step into the world of the employed. Most of us have more than one career. Actually, the average is more like three or four major changes in career direction in the course of our work life.

Preparation for the Job Hunt

Many books and articles have been written about the content and process of job hunting. The very volume of this literature should suggest the extent to which it is a common problem for North Americans. Most of us are amateur job hunters because we spend most of our adult life working, not looking for work. To the novice hunter, looking for work often seems a special form of agony. Job hunting can be a predictably positive experience given a positive attitude, the correct tools, a supportive environment, and some maturity in planning and information-seeking techniques.

A Positive Attitude

"I'm sure I'll never get a job, I don't have any experience or training, nobody wants to hire someone with epilepsy." This is not the attitude with which to begin. It's common among young adults and it has a self-defeating truth to it the more it is repeated. The young adult who has had many years of being a contributing family member and who has had meaningful feedback on his performance for years or who views learning as an opportunity, has a more positive option . . . "I'm pretty sure I'll get a job because I know I'm a hard worker—I've mowed the lawn and taken care of our car for years. I haven't done paid work but I listen well and I'll do my job just the way my boss wants it done. I know that employers have a hard time finding steady, reliable people and I can offer that." That's positive! This child may need help to rehearse it, but it works!

The Correct Tools

The tools of the job hunt are being able to read a newspaper, use a telephone directory, fill out application forms, write a resume, get around town without losing direction in time for the interviews, basic communication skills, and the ability to tell the nice and skillful things about oneself. People with epilepsy must face the application form and the job interview differently than nondisabled job hunters. While human rights legislation varies from country to country and from state to state, most application forms ask about any chronic medical condition that might limit the applicant's ability to perform the job. The person with epilepsy has four choices in responding: Leaving that space blank; lying and denying any such condition; writing in "epilepsy" or "seizure disorder"; filling in "will discuss at interview."

While each person must make a personal decision on which choice to use, there are some considerations for and against. If the space is left blank, one can be reasonably sure the form won't immediately be thrown into the wastebasket but the interviewer will ask the applicant to respond. So, an explanation must be ready. If one chooses to lie by blatantly denying the existence of the epilepsy, that individual may get past that possible point of discrimination but a reasonable cause for dismissal is also provided if the lie is uncovered later. Of course, the applicant can lie on the form and correct it at the interview, in which case the interviewer may be sympathetic or simply annoyed. If "epilepsy" or "seizure disorder" is written in, full marks are given for honesty and a possible filing in the wastebasket. On the other hand, some people understand the employment difficulties of disabled individuals. The fourth alternative "will discuss at interview" is not a lie, neither is it a guarantee that the interviewer will suddenly become uncontrollably curious about the explanation. Everyone has their personal opinion about the best strategy. The risks of the first and last alternatives seem most preferable.

The job interview holds a special challenge for persons with epilepsy. Those who maintain they experience unfair discrimination as soon as they mention the word *epilepsy* frequently dwell on how much or how little to say about their condition. Again, there are choices to think over; then, the response should be rehearsed until the person feels comfortable. Some examples of responses are given below.

Short and to the point: "I have epilepsy, a medical condition for which I am receiving medical care and which I believe does not affect my ability to work."

Long-winded and usually overly technical: "I have a medical condition called epilepsy. This means that approximately once every month I have a generalized seizure (or whichever type applies). I have a reliable aura beforehand and my loss of consciousness lasts only (approximately) minutes. My recovery time after a seizure varies, but I feel I could responsibly perform my duties."

To the point and relevant to the job setting: "I have epilepsy. I don't know if you are familiar with this medical condition but I think I should tell you a little about my seizures. On my last job, I had three seizures all the time I worked there. Altogether, I guess they took up about the time it takes for three coffeebreaks. I was at my last job for 2 years. By telling my co-workers what to do in case of a seizure they felt comfortable around me. Since I am receiving medical treatment, I am just as capable of doing my job well as anyone else, who for example, requires glasses for poor eyesight. Would you like to ask me any questions about epilepsy?''

Which method would assist the employer the most in assessing whether epilepsy should prevent someone from getting a job? Which approach would help the most when one has to make a judgment about an applicant's ability to work, and to communicate well enough with the co-workers to fit in? If the interviewers were doctors, but even if they are not, the second choice would probably be the clearest. If the equivalent of two, six, or even twelve coffee breaks is considered an insignificant loss of time due to illness or injury over a 2-year period (it would be great if all employees could be so healthy!), obviously the third approach works the best. Individuals with epilepsy often receive advice from neurologists, epileptologists, and their team members regarding realistic employment. In addition to letters, physicians may be requested to contact the company doctor especially if there is resistance to hire a person with epilepsy on unjustified medical grounds.

A Supportive Environment

Looking for work alone can be frustrating and lonely. With a group of other job hunters, it can become a positive and supportive experience. Local employment centers, community colleges, and continuing education programs often carry time-limited, curriculum-based job hunt courses. These should be investigated. Buddying up with a friend and buying a short "how to" book on job hunting can be very helpful. Most book stores have a business section where such literature can be found. The local librarian can also assist. Former school counselors are usually willing and eager to see students return for advice. The hardest part of the job hunt is not gathering the tools for it, nor those interviews with sweaty palms and dry throats, but the in-between times spent searching for new leads. This is where positive support is needed. The most effective job hunts (how long it takes to find work and how rewarding it is financially and otherwise) are the intensive and systematic group efforts that involve several hours every day. In short, it should be treated as a full time job!

Parents can help by providing practical leads. They can supply a name, address, and phone number of a contact (not a good friend) who would not mind talking with the child. Parents could offer some of their chore time if they are confident that this would be appreciated. They might free up the family telephone if calls are expected and they could rehearse the interview setting with their children as a method of reducing anxiety. Parents shouldn't manufacture an unneeded job for them due to a belief that a "real" one won't ever be found. If that is the feeling, the community resources for job training and for sheltered employment need to be explored and discussed. There are several ways of obtaining job training in most larger communities:

On-the-job training -provided by business, industry, and rehabilitation centers

Apprenticeship programs sponsored by industry, unions, and government

Community college and technical institute programs

University programs

School or government work

Experience or activity programs that lead to job placement.

Sheltered employment refers to special job sites or to adapted employment, which caters to some of the disabled population. Not everyone can work competitively in a society that operates by profit motives; some are capable of eventual competitive employment but may need a gradual immersion into the work world. Although we all need meaning to our lives to feel useful, not all of us define usefulness as being equivalent to earning power. Not everyone has their set of unique capabilities developed at an even level. Some of us are efficient workers when presented with a task, but can't decide on our own which task to take on next. Some people need more supervision in a work setting than is available in the competitive labor market.

Unfortunately, many more people are in sheltered industries than need to be. When well-intentioned persons suggest such an alternative, parents and the young adult should visit that particular facility. Industries where employees are busy and their work pattern is meaningful are potentially healthy environments. Here much can be learned and taught.

Maturity in Planning and Organizing Skills

The process of looking for employment is most effective when it is preceded by thoughtful planning. Organization of materials and methods are required to effectively follow-up on job leads. An employer is not impressed with a smudged resume or erratically filled-out application forms. Many individuals with epilepsy who encounter significant difficulties in locating employment lack basic organizing skills. Most of us organize gradually and without instruction, by modeling what have appeared to us to be effective procedures. Some children may not have learned these principles spontaneously, thus a structure may be of great help in getting them to efficiently search for work. There are some practical guidelines:

> There should be an "office" area in the child's bedroom. This may be a desk with a cardboard box for filing paper away such as sample application forms, copies of his resume, lists of people to contact the next day, copies of letters already sent, etc. Strict office hours should be organized. Interview and contact times are set. A spiral bound pocket-sized notebook or a spiral bound index cards should be purchased. On it, the places of interviews, contacts, addresses, and phone numbers of employment centers are recorded, with a daily diary of job hunting activities. Different sized envelopes and stamps should be on hand with a calendar and an office time table. Short positive interludes should be arranged in the time-table (coffee break).

When parents are helping their "job hunters" to set up an "office," they should not impose their system of organization until it is established that it is the most sensible for the job hunter. Otherwise, parents will have to be around constantly to retrieve materials. For example, a parent may file alphabetically but the young adult has a fantastic memory and organizes easiest by putting things away in the order they were received (by time/number). Or, one may organize left to right but another does it right to left. Again, it is ideal to hunt for jobs with a buddy or in a group so perhaps two or three friends in a similar unemployed state could set up a joint office in a basement. For each interview, the job hunter should carry a folder that contains two copies of the resume, letters of reference, information already collected on the company, and paper to write down thoughts and plans that were discussed.

Maintaining and Moving Up in Jobs

Because career development is a process, it implies constant movement. Getting employment does not guarantee continuance and even if it is maintained, sameness can eventually lead to boredom. A positive attitude toward both self and the work world is the safeguard against stagnation. Job interests do not even begin to come firmly together into a pattern until the mid-twenties, so the chances of a first employment being the only one are few. Moving up career ladders seems to be an expectation of most of us because society puts much emphasis on achievement through our work identities.

When finally work is found it may be so much of a relief for the job hunter and the family that everyone needs and deserves a period of stability. Maintaining and moving up, however, are as important as the earlier phases. People with epilepsy are especially concerned with keeping their employment because many are dismissed after having one or two seizures during work. These unfortunate events are often presented as a catastrophe that took only seconds to transpire. This is often not the case. It may have been the first time a convulsion was witnessed in that job and that the person with epilepsy did not discuss it with the employer. Ignoring such episodes, however, is not a good strategy because it leaves everyone uncertain of what to expect next, what caused it, and so on. Simple questions and hidden fears must be brought into the open, at least with the boss. If a person is fired for attempting to talk about the seizure afterward, he or she probably would have been dismissed anyway.

Summary of the Career Development Process

The process of preparing for adult employment is one that begins early in life and continues as long as the individual is involved in the work world. This process is one of gradual development through phases of fantasy, emerging career awareness and education, exploration into different types of work activity with tentative commitments being made to different careers. The gradual development of decision-making or problem-solving skills facilitates the phase of formal commitment to a job. People generally make more than one significant and formal career decision in the course of their working lives.

The process of career development and maturity is predictable. Therefore, our educational institutions have been able to come up with programs that meet the career needs of students in different phases.

Many people with epilepsy experience stumbling blocks in their job preparation activities. Some of these are discrimination on the part of employers, over-simplification of the job-hunting process, inadequate education of others about epilepsy, poorly developed planning or organizing abilities and decision-making skills, insufficient knowledge about self and the world of work, and the lack of proper work attitudes. Many of these stumbling blocks are avoidable, and all can be removed or alleviated.

Where to Go for Help

Families who wish to know more about epilepsy services could call their physicians, the nearest Seizure Clinics or the local Epilepsy Societies. Additionally, in the United States, the Epilepsy Foundation of America (EFA) provides comprehensive information (1828 L Street, N.W., Suite 406, Washington, D.C. 20036).

In Canada, the Canadian League Against Epilepsy (Health Sciences Centre Hospital, 2075 Wesbrook Place, U.B.C. Campus, Vancouver, B.C. V6Y 1W5) could be contacted.

The EFA is a national organization that is strongly committed to the Epilepsy movement. They are a major contributor to both medical and public understanding of epilepsy. They provide pamphlets, reprints, books, films, and statistics on seizure disorders, continuously updated lists of educational materials for families and teachers, information on insurances, pharmacy services, epilepsy programs, and even on fund raising and the legal rights of individuals with seizures. Parents of children with epilepsy should subscribe to the official Newsletter of EFA, the National Spokesman.

Afterword

The writing of this book was an arduous task. Complex medical issues were translated into everyday language so that parents and older children with seizures could understand them. We tried to avoid becoming overly simple or complex, and included just enough information on the most important aspects of epilepsy. Scientific terms commonly used by doctors were explained throughout the text. These could not be eliminated. Our opinions may differ from that of some but we believe the majority of practicing physicians share our approach. If any of the readers have suggestions for the second edition on how to improve the presentation of the various topics, perhaps they could let us know.

Index

Absence seizures, *see* Petit mal seizures
Activated charcoal, for overdose, 141
Addiction, to anticonvulsants, 115–117
Adolescents, *see* Teenagers
Air bubble test, *see* Pneumoencephalogram
Airplane travel, 160
Akinetic seizure, in secondary generalized epilepsy, 77
Alcohol, 179, 180
Allergic reactions, to specific medications, 128–129
Ambulance, seizures requiring, 152
Anger, in families, 169–170
Angiogram, 46, 47
Anticonvulsants, *see* Drug therapy
Application forms, for employment, 212–213
Astatic seizure, in secondary generalized epilepsy, 77
Atonic seizure, 87
  in secondary generalized epilepsy, 77
Atypical absence spells, *see* Secondary generalized epilepsy
Atypical febrile seizure, *see* Complex febrile seizure
Aura, 86
  in partial epilepsy, 69
Automatisms, in petit mal seizures, 55

Babysitting, for child with epilepsy, 158

Barbiturates, 62, 132–133
Bathing, for child with epilepsy, 159–160
Behavioral problems, 196–197
Behavioral treatment approaches, 139–140
Benign Sylvian seizures of childhood, 70
Blood levels
  drug discontinuance and, 110
  of drugs, 106–108
  medication schedules and, 111
Blood tests, 45–46
Boxing, for child with epilepsy, 177
Bracelets, identifying, 158–159
Brain
  examining, *see* Tests
  formation of, 13, 14
  location of fundamental functions of, 14–18, 85–87
  neurological examinations and, 34–35
  surgery, 138–139
Brain abscess, 22
Brain damage, 6, 192, 193
  seizures causing, 24–25
Brain dysfunction, 6, 192
  learning difficulties caused by, 193
Brain stem, 17, 18
Brain tumor, seizures caused by, 21
Brain wave test (electroencephalogram), *see* Tests
Brand name of drugs, 119
Breastfeeding, by mother with epilepsy, 182
Breath-holding spells, 99
Bromide, 9

Camping, for child with epilepsy, 177
Canadian League Against Epilepsy, 219
Car, taking long trips in, 160
  see also Driving
Carbamezepine, see Tegretol
Career preparation, see Employment
CAT scan, 43–45
Causes of epilepsy, 20–22
Celontin, 131, 132, 135
Central nervous system
  disorders, 22
  formation of the, 13, 14
  see also Brain
Cerebellum, 17
  abnormal, 35
Cerebral palsy, 195–196
Cerebro-spinal fluid, 46
Cerebrum, 14, 15, 16, 17
Chains, identifying, 158–159
Childhood
  career preparation and, 206–209
  effect of epilepsy in, 166–168
Childhood illnesses
  immunizations for, 157–158
  seizures during, 157
Clonic phase, of grand mal seizures, 61, 62
Clonopin, 111, 131, 132, 135, 136
Complex partial seizures, see Partial
  seizures
Complex febrile seizures, 42, 92–93
Computerized axial tomography, see
  CAT scan
Concussion, 22
Consciousness, 151
  during a seizure, 151–152
Constipation in infancy, seizures
  and, 24
Contact sports, for child with
  epilepsy, 177
Conversion table, from metric
  measurements, 130
Convulsion
  definition, 19
  management of child during, 8,
  147–154
  see also Grand mal seizures;
  Seizures
Convulsive attacks, 53
  see also Grand mal seizures

Corpus callosum, 14, 15, 18
Cortex, 14, 15, 86–87
Cryptogenic epilepsy, see Idiopathic
  epilepsy

Dating, for teenager with epilepsy,
  179–181
Daydreaming, 97
Deep breathing, see Hyperventilation
Dental hygiene, Dilantin and, 118,
  119, 131
Depakene, 53, 93, 106, 111, 131,
  132, 134
Developmental delay, see Brain
  dysfunction
Developmental stages, effects of
  epilepsy and, 166–168
Diagnosis
  parental views on, 3
  second medical opinion and,
  121–122
Diamox, 131, 132, 136
Diazepines, 135–136
Diets, 137
  ketogenic, 140
Dilantin, 9, 105–106, 107, 113, 131
  alcohol and, 179
  gum hypertrophy and, 118, 119,
  131
  initial dose of, 109
  pregnancy and, 181
  side effects of, 130–131, 132
Diones, 136
Disability, 8
Discipline, for the multihandicapped,
  198–201
Doctor, see Physician
Dose-dependent side effects, 128
Double dose, 112
Drinking (alcohol), 179–180
Driving, 177–179
  insurance for, 183
  light-sensitive seizures in, 64, 66
  long trips in car and, 161
  teenagers and, 117, 177–179
Drug therapy
  addiction to, 115–117
  barbiturates, 62, 132–133
  carbamezepine, 131, 133–134, 181
  for complex febrile seizures, 93

for complex partial seizures, 72
diazepines, 135–136
discontinuing, 110–111, 117–118
double dosage, 112
electroencephalogram and, 39
in emergency, 153–154
failure of, 136–140
frequency of administration, 111,
    111–112, 113, 114
for grand mal seizures, 62
gum hypertrophy and, 118, 119,
    131
head trauma and, 22
hydantoins, 130–132
for infantile spasms, 80
initial dose, 127
interactions, 106, 157
learning difficulties caused by, 194
in liquid form, 112–115, 143
maintenance dose and, 106–108
mechanisms of, 105–106
metric measurements of, 129–130
noncompliance, 111–112, 113, 114
overdosage, 141–142
parents administering, 153–154
for petit mal seizures, 55–56,
    58–59
pharmacies and, 118–120
in pill form, 112, 115, 142–143
in school situation, 161
for secondary generalized
    epilepsy, 77
seizures due to, 24
selection of, 127
side effects, 127–129, 130–136
starting, 108–110
storage, 136
succinimides, 135
Tegretol, 131, 133–134, 181
uncooperative child and, 142–143
valproic acid, 134
see also Prescription drugs;
    specific drugs

Early childhood, *see* Preschoolers
Educable mental retardation, 195
Education for All Handicapped Chil-
    dren Act (Public Law 94–142),
    184
see also School

EEG (electroencephalogram), *see*
    Tests
Electroencephalogram (EEG), *see*
    Tests
Electroencephalography, 9
Elementary school years, career pre-
    paration and, 207–209
Emergencies, drug administration
    during, 153–154
Emotions, *see* Feelings
Employment
    discrimination in, 184, 205
    job hunting, 212–215, 216
    maintaining and moving up in,
        216–217
    planning and organizing skills
        for, 216
    preparation for, 205, 217–218
        early childhood and, 206–207
        elementary school and, 207–209
        junior high school and, 209–211
        secondary school and, 211
    training, 215
    sheltered, 215
Encephalitis, 8, 22
Encephalopathy, secondary general-
    ized epilepsy and, 75–76
Epilepsy
    definition, 18
    misconceptions about, 6–9
    origin of term, 9
Epilepsy clinics nurses, 185–186
Epilepsy Foundation of America
    (EFA), 183, 219
    Pharmacy Service of, 120
Epilepsy Societies, 219
Epileptic attack, *see* Seizure
Epileptologists, 33
Evaporated milk, for overdose, 141
Examination, *see* Medical
    examination

Fainting, 97–98
Family
    feelings of, 168–170
    lay epilepsy organizations for,
        183–184
    of multihandicapped child, 190
    as network, 173
    see also Parents; Siblings
Family physician, 33

Fatigue, avoidance of, 62
  see also Sleep
Fear, grand mal seizure and,
    62–63, 150
Febrile seizures, 24, 91–94, 149
  complex, 42, 92–93
  heredity and, 182–183
  phenobarbital and, 108
  simple, 42, 92, 93
Fecal incontinence, grand mal
    seizure and, 61
Feelings
  childhood and, 166–168
  of family, 168–170
  of parents, 4, 170–171
  of siblings, 172–173
Fever
  during convulsion, 149
  immunizations causing, 157–158
  see also Febrile seizures
Focal seizures, see Partial seizures
Football, for child with epilepsy, 177
Frontal lobe, 14, 15, 16, 17
  complex partial seizures originat-
    ing from, 71

Generalized seizure, 19, 87
  sleeping arrangements and, 159
Generic name of drug, 119
Genetic counseling, 181, 182–183
Genetic factors, see Heredity
Grand mal seizures, 53, 60–62,
    76, 87
  definition, 19
  fear managed in, 62–63, 150
  management of child during, 8,
    147–154
  stages of, 61–62
  traveling and, 160
  uncertainty managed in, 63–64,
    165–166
Grey matter, 14, 15
  see also Cortex
Group Life Insurance Plan of
    Epilepsy Foundation of
    America, 183
Guilt
  after convulsion, 150
  in families, 169–170
  in parents, 4

Gum hypertrophy, Dilantin and,
    118, 119, 131

Hallucinogenic drugs, 179
Handedness, development of, 17–18
Handicap, 8
  epilepsy as an invisible, 8–9
"Hard" neurological signs, 35
Headache
  after grand mal seizure, 62, 150
  migraine, 95–96
Head trauma
  contact sports and, 177
  epilepsy caused by, 21–22
Hearing loss, 196
Heart attacks, epilepsy confused
    with, 8
Helmets, physical injury protection
    by, 141, 142
Helplessness, in families, 169–170
Hemiplegic migraine, 95
Hemispheres of brain, 14–17
Heredity, 21, 53, 182–183
  benign Sylvian seizures of child-
    hood and, 70
  primary generalized convulsions
    and, 62
High school, career preparation
    and, 211
  see also Teenagers
Hippocrates, 9
Historical viewpoints, on epilepsy,
    9–10
History taking
  physician and, 33–34, 72
  for hospital, 48
Hockey, for child with epilepsy, 177
Hospitalization, 47–50
  seizure requiring, 152–153
Hydantoins, 130–132
Hyperactivity, 194–195
  partial seizures and, 73
  from phenobarbital, 133
  myoclonic-absence seizure and,
    84–85
Hyperventilation, petit mal
    seizures and, 37
Hypnogogic jerks, 94
Hypsarrhythmic pattern, in infantile
    spasms, 78–79
Hysterical seizures, 53

Identifying bracelets, 158–159
Identifying chains, 158–159
Idiopathic epilepsy, 21, 86
Idiopathic generalized epilepsy, *see*
    Primary (idiopathic) general-
    ized epilepsy
Idiopathic generalized tonic-clonic
    convulsions, heredity and,
    182–183
Immunizations, 157–158
Incidence of epilepsy, 5–6
Incomplete absence spells, *see*
    Secondary generalized epilepsy
Infancy
    infantile spasms in, 77–80, 117
    mothers having epilepsy and,
        181–182
    seizures in, 24
    startle response in, 94
Infantile spasms, 77–80, 117
Insurance, for individuals with
    epilepsy, 183
Intercoms, 159
Intermittent photic stimulation,
    photosensitive epilepsy
    and, 37
International League Against
    Epilepsy, 53
Intoxications, epilepsy caused
    by, 22
Intramuscular injections, parents
    administering, 153–154
Ipecac, for overdose, 141

Jack-knife convulsions, *see*
    Infantile spasms
Jacksonian March, *see* Somatosen-
    sory partial seizures
Jerks, 97
Job hunting, 212–215, 216
    see also Employment
Job interview, 213–214
Junior high school, career prepara-
    tion and, 209–211

Ketogenic diet, for myoclonic
    seizures, 137–138, 140

Labels, multihandicapped and,
    192–193
Language delay, 196
Lay Epilepsy Organizations,
    183–184
Learning disabilities, 193–194
Left hemisphere, 16–17
Lennox-Gastaut syndrome, 80,
    81–83, 117
Light-sensitive seizures, *see*
    Photosensitive seizures
Limbic cortex, 16
Limbic lobe, 15
Limits, for the multihandicapped,
    198–201
Liquid, as drug format, 112–115, 143
Low seizure threshold, 42
Luminal, 131, 132

Maintenance dose of drugs, 106–108
    therapy started with a, 108–109
Marriage, 7, 181
    genetic counseling, 182–183
    pregnancy and, 181–182
Massive myoclonic jerks, *see*
    Infantile spasms
MCT oil, 137
Mebaral, 131, 132
Medic Alert, 159
Medical examination
    history taking in, 33–34
    neurological examination, 34–35
    see also Tests
Medical information, parents
    needing, 4
Medications, *see* Drug therapy
Medium chain trygliceride, 137
Meningitis, 8, 22
Mental illness, 7
Mental retardation, 6–7, 189–190,
    195
Mesantoin, 131, 132
Metabolism
    of drugs, 107–108
    screening for, 105–106
Metric system, for dose measure-
    ments, 129–130
Middle childhood, reaction to
    epilepsy and, 167–168
Migraine headache, 95–96

Milk, for drug overdose, 141
Milontin, 131, 132, 135
Minimal brain dysfunction, 192–193
Misconceptions, about epilepsy,
     6–9
Mogadon, 131, 132, 136
Mouth
   placement of objects in, 149
   tongue swallowing and, 7–8,
     62, 148
Multidisciplinary team approach,
     122, 191–192
Multihandicapped child
   behavioral problems in, 196–197
   burden of on family, 189–190
   cerebral palsy in, 195–196
   diagnosis after birth, 190–191
   hearing loss in, 196
   hyperactivity in, 194–195
   labels and, 192–193
   learning disabilities in, 193–194
   limits used for, 198–201
   mental retardation in, 189–190,
     195
   parents and, 5
   speech and language delay in, 196
   team approach for, 122, 191–192
   visual impairment in, 196
Myoclonic-absence seizures, 84–85
Myoclonic seizure, 97
   ketogenic diet for, 137–138
   in secondary generalized epilepsy,
     77
Mysoline, 131, 132, 133

Nasopharyngeal leads, 37
National Spokesman, 219
Neurological examination, 34–35
Neurologist, 33
Neuroradiological techniques, 138
Neurosurgery, 138
Night terrors, 94
Nocturnal seizures, 24, 159
   in secondary generalized epilepsy,
     76–77
Noncompliance, drug therapy and,
     111–112, 113–114
Nonconvulsive attacks, 53
   see also Petit mal seizures

Nonspecific abnormality, electro-
     encephalogram and, 41
Nurses, for epilepsy clinics, 185–186

Occipital lobe, 14, 16, 17
   seizures originating from, see
     Special sensory seizures
Overdosage, 141–142
Oxygen
   lack of at birth, 22
   parental administration of, 153

Pallid syncope, 98–99
Paradione, 131, 132, 136
Paraldehyde, rectal administration
     of, 153, 160
Parents
   advice to other parents from, 5
   attitudes of toward child with
     epilepsy, 3–4
   child with epilepsy viewed by, 4–5
   communication by with health
     providers, 185–186
   diagnosis of epilepsy and, 3
   doctor and
     appointments, 122–123
     relationship with, 33
   effect of child with epilepsy on,
     170–171
   guilt feelings of, 4
   intramuscular medications admin-
     istered by, 153–154
   job hunt assistance from, 215, 216
   management of child with convul-
     sions by, 147–154
   management of child with partial
     seizures by, 73–74
   marriage of and the child with
     epilepsy, 5
   medical information needed for, 4
   reactions of to the seizures,
     166–167
     first seizure, 22–24, 147
     petit mal seizures, 57
   school for child and, 4
   severely multihandicapped child
     and, 5
   starter book for children and,
     26–29

see also Family
Parietal lobe, 14-15, 16
Paroxysmal activity, electroenceph-
    alogram and, 42
Partial seizures, 19, 61, 87
  benign Sylvian seizures of child-
      hood, 70
  complex, 55, 70-74
    parental intervention during,
        147-148
    electroencephalogram for, 69
    origin of symptoms and signs in,
        53, 54
    parents managing, 73-74
    somatosensory, 74-75
    special sensory, 75
Parties, teenage years and, 179, 180
Patient's Bill of Rights, 184
Pediatrician, 33
Pediatric neurologist, 33
Petit mal seizures, 19, 53-56, 62
  child and
    information to about seizure,
        59-60
    medication and feelings of,
        58-59
  drug therapy for, 55-56, 58-59
  electroencephalogram of, 41, 55
  heredity and, 182-183
  hyperventilation and, 37
  learning difficulties caused by,
      193-194
  parental reactions to, 57
Pharmacies, 118-120
Phenobarbital, 106, 132
  pregnancy and, 181
  febrile seizures and, 93, 94, 108
Photosensitive epilepsy, 24, 64-66
  heredity and, 182-183
  intermittent photic stimulation
      and, 37
Physician
  choosing a, 33
  communicating with, 185-186
  information about seizure
      requested by, 151-152
  parents going to appointments of,
      122-123
  second medical opinion and,
      121-122
  seizure requiring, 152-153

see also Medical examination
Pills, as drug format, 112, 115,
    142-143
Pneumoencephalogram, 46-47
Post-ictal state, of grand mal
    seizures, 61-62, 150
Post-traumatic epilepsy, 22
Pregnancy
  epilepsy caused by factors in, 20
  in women with epilepsy, 181-182
    breastfeeding and, 182
  see also Heredity
Preschoolers
  career preparation and, 206-207
  effects of epilepsy on, 166-167
  informed about epilepsy, 25-26
Prescription drugs, 120-121
  abbreviations, 120, 121
  pharmacies and, 118-120
  prescriptions and, 120-121
  see also Drug therapy
Primary (idiopathic) generalized
    epilepsy, 21, 62, 86
  see also Grand mal seizures; Petit
    mal seizures; Photosensitive
    epilepsy
Prognosis, 37
Protective helmets, 141, 142
Pseudo-seizures, *see* Psychogenic
    epilepsy
Psychogenic epilepsy, 99-101
Public Law 94-142 (Education for
    All Handicapped Children
    Act), 184
  see also School

Quack advice, 140

Recreation, for child with
    epilepsy, 177
Rectally administered medications,
    153-154, 160
Reflex vagal syncope, *see* Pallid
    syncope
Right hemisphere, 16-17
Rights of children with epilepsy, 184
Ritalin, 161
Rivotril, *see* Clonopin
Rules, for the multihandicapped,
    198-201

Sadness, in families, 169–170
Salaam seizures, *see* Infantile
    spasms
School, 160–162
    buddy system at, 177
    career preparation and, 207–211
    hospital provision for, 49
Secondary generalized epilepsy,
    75–77
    electroencephalogram in, 77
    infantile spasms, 77–80
    Lennox-Gestaut syndrome, 80,
        81–93, 117
    myoclonic-absence seizures, 84–85
Secondary school, career preparation
    and, 211
Second medical opinion, 121–122
Seizures
    brain abnormality and, 85–87
    brain damage and, 24–25
    causes of the, 20–22, 24
    definition, 18, 19, 37
    during childhood illnesses, 157
    during electroencephalogram,
        39, 41
    during pregnancy, 181
    immunizing a child who has,
        157–158
    important observations during a,
        151–152
    learning difficulties caused by,
        193–194
    management of child during,
        147–154
    marriage and social life of parents
        and, 5
    reactions to first, 22–24, 47,
        166–167
    sleeping arrangements and, 159
    see also Generalized seizure;
        Grand mal seizures; Partial
        seizures; Petit mal seizures
Seizure disorder, 19
Seizure clinics, 33, 219
Severely multihandicapped child,
    parents' views on, 5
    see also Multihandicapped child
Sheltered employment, 215
Showering, for child with epilepsy,
    160
Siblings
    anger of, 169

epilepsy in, 183
    feelings of, 170, 172–173
    medical examination and, 34
Side effects of drugs, 127–129
Simple febrile convulsions, 42,
    92–93
Skull x-rays, 43
Sleep
    arrangements for, 159
    deprivation of for electroencepha-
        logram, 38, 69
    following convulsion, 61–62,
        149–150
    night terrors, 94
    twitches during, 94
    see also Nocturnal seizures
Smoking, 179, 180
"Soft" neurological signs, 35
Somatosensory partial seizures,
    74–75
Special sensory seizures, 75
Speech disturbance, 196
Sphenoidal electrode, 37
Spinal cord, systems in, 87
Spinal tap, 46
Sports, 177
Starter book, for parents and chil-
    dren, 26–29
Startling, 94
Status epilepticus, 25, 111
Steady state, of drug and, 107, 108
Strokes, 22
Succinimides, 135
Summer camps, 177
Surgery, 138–139
Swimming, 159
Syncope
    fainting, 97–98
    pallid, 98–99

Tantrums, temper, 96–97
Team approach, for multihandi-
    capped, 191–192
Teenagers
    career preparation and
        in high school, 211
        in junior high school, 209–211
    dating, 179–181
    discontinuance of drug therapy
        and, 117
    driving and, 117, 177–179

hospitalization of, 49
light-sensitive seizures in, 64, 66
medical examination and, 34
noncompliance and, 112, 113
parties attended by, 179, 180
pregnancy among, 181
reaction to epilepsy by, 167–168
responsibility of for taking medica-
    tion, 58, 111, 112, 113
Tegretol and, 133–134
Teething, seizures and, 24
Tegretol, 131, 132, 133–134
pregnancy and, 181
Temper tantrums, 96–97
Temporal lobe, 17
complex partial seizures originat-
    ing from the, 55, 70–71, 72–73,
    96–97
Temporal lobe epilepsy, 55, 70–71,
    72–73, 96–97
Tests
angiogram, 46, 47
of blood, 45–46
CAT scan, 43–45
electroencephalogram
    discontinuing medication
        and, 117
    in infantile spasms, 78–79
    in secondary generalized
        epilepsy, 77
    in Lennox-Gastaut syndrome,
        82–83
    in partial epilepsy, 69
    in primary generalized
        seizure, 53
    in petit mal seizure, 55
pneumoencephalogram, 46–47
skull x-rays, 43
spinal tap, 46
Tics, 97
Todd's paralysis, 150
Tongue
biting, 61
swallowing, 7–8, 62, 148
Tonic-clonic seizure, idiopathic
    generalized, 182–183
see also Grand mal seizure
Tonic phase, of grand mal seizures,
    61, 62
Tonic seizure, 77, 87
Toxicity, dosage and, 106
Trainable mental retardation, 195

Tranxene, 131, 132, 136
Traveling, for child with
    epilepsy, 160
Treatment
behavioral approaches, 139, 140
ketogenic diet, 137–138, 140
protective helmets, 141
quack advice, 140
surgery, 138–139
see also Drug therapy
Tridione, 131, 132, 136
Trips, for child with epilepsy, 160
Tuberous scherosis, infantile spasms
    and, 80

Uncertainties, in epilepsy, 63–64,
    165–166
Uncooperative child, medications
    given to an, 142–143
Urinary incontinence, grand mal
    seizure and, 61

Valium, 131, 132, 133, 135
rectal administration of, 153,
    154, 160
Valproic acid, 134
Visual impairment, 196
Vocation, see Employment
Vocational Rehabilitation Act of
    1973, 184
Vomiting
during convulsion, 7, 148
from childhood illness, 157
migraine headache and, 95

Walking, 72
see also Complex partial seizures
WEP, see Work education/experi-
    ence programs
White matter, see Corpus callosum
Work, see Employment
Work education/experience programs
    (WEP), 210–211
Wrestling, 177

X-rays, of skull, 43

Zarontin, 131, 132, 135
for petit mal seizure, 55, 56